Avoiding Atherosclerosis

Avoiding Atherosclerosis

A Scientific Approach to Eating

RONALD L. WATHEN, M.D., Ph.D., FACP
CURTIS L. BARRETT, Ph.D., ABPP

ORANGE *frazer* PRESS
Wilmington, Ohio

Published for Ronald Wathen and Curtis Barrett by:
Orange Frazer Press
P.O. Box 214
Wilmington, OH 45177
Telephone 1.800.852.9332 for price and shipping information.
Website: www.orangefrazer.com
www.orangefrazercustombooks.com

Book and cover design: Brittany Lament and Orange Frazer Press

Library of Congress Control Number: 2012949464

This book is dedicated to my parents, Margaret and Lowell Wathen. My father died of an acute MI at age 73 and my mother died of a series of strokes at age 80, both complications of atherosclerosis. They were the finest parents one could have. I think of them daily.

—Ron Wathen

My efforts in this book are dedicated to my father, Curtis Leo Barrett, Sr., and to my brother, Frank W. Barrett, who were lost while so very young to atherosclerosis; and also to my mother, Ina R. Barrett Gardner, whose love and genes have allowed me the time to understand why this happened to them.

—Curtis Barrett

Table of Contents

Section Two

Epilogue   145

Appendices

Index   155

Foreword

Very often, books such as this are written following a passionate working life of intensive research and clinical caring. This book is like that. The authors, experienced in the rigor of scientific investigation and scientific journal writing, are now at the point where they can express what's in their guts after all those years of constraint. We now feel free to speak plainly to those who want to listen.

Also, books such as this often have a story behind them. That too is a characteristic of this book. The story began when the authors were about eight years old, a few months shy of beginning second grade in a rural, southern Indiana township. Ron was lying on a daybed, on his porch, reading a Superman comic book when Curt appeared at his door in tears, lost and terrified. He had become lost in his new neighborhood while taking a bucket of grapes to his aunt, who lived a short distance from Ron. Curt had made one of the many wrong turns of his life while not paying enough attention to his surroundings.

Ron called his mother for help and she knew just how to calm a crying little boy and send him in the right direction for home. Actually, he was barely a mile away from home, as the crow flies, but he was thoroughly lost. Later, in the fall, Ron and Curt became classmates and continued that way through grade school and high school. Although, in high school, they didn't "run" in the same crowd, they have remained close friends ever since. In college, Ron began what was to become a career in science and medicine. Curt embarked on a career in the Navy via the Regular NROTC.

It is fair to say that an early love of science changed the life of both Ron and Curt. Ron was accepted into the M.D./Ph.D. combined degree program at Indiana University, Bloomington. After completing his Ph.D., he did a year's research fellowship in Renal Physiology at the I.U. Medical Center in Indianapolis and after this, transferred to the Southwestern Medical Center/U of TX, Dallas, to complete his M.D. degree. Ron did his inital post-graduate medical training at Parkland Hospital in Dallas, TX, and the VAMC in Dallas, TX, and completed his post-graduate training at Vanderbilt University Hospital in Nashville, TN. After college, Curt was assigned to a ship that did research on anti-submarine devices in addition to the work of a regular destroyer. When it became clear that the research was poorly designed, and did not take into account human factors, Curt left the Navy, intending to return after finishing a degree in Human Engineering. Later Curt changed careers again and became a Ph.D. Clinical Psychologist, at the University of Louisville School of Medicine, doing research and treatment mainly in the field of addictions and Cognitive Behavioral Therapy. He remained in the Naval Reserve for over 30 more years. Curt, like Ron, was never far from scientific inquiry while practicing in an academic setting.

Both Ron and Curt achieved international reputations in their fields and, of all things, eventually became professors in the same medical school. It was in the latter role that they renewed the friendship that began when Curt was a little boy, surrounded by "lostness," and rescued by Ron's mother.

Ron's career also took twists and turns over the years. His scientific work began as he pursued the Ph.D. in Physiology, received that degree, and continued on his way to the M.D. Armed with these two advanced degrees, he chose the field of kidney disease and became a nephrologist. Ron's career in academic medicine, which included the practical tasks of directing clinical services and supervising aspiring nephrologists, spanned about 30 years. He published extensively and remained faithful to his Ph.D.'s admonition to contribute new knowledge to his field.

There was another twist and turn. Ron decided to find out what private practice was all about. To this end, he left academia and moved to a small town in Southwestern Ohio. This move had a very important effect on Ron's thinking and his practice. It provided a very homogenous, primarily caucasian, population for study and to care for. And, for the first time, Ron became profoundly interested in atherosclerosis or hardening of the arteries and, in particular, how overweight, obesity, and diabetes played such major roles in furthering atherosclerosis.

So, the story now questions how two 76–year–old, mostly retired, former classmates in grade school came to be collaborators in the study of atherosclerosis. We find another twist here. After his retirement, when Curt suffered a stroke while in Africa, Ron came to see him as soon as he returned home. Although the focus was on teaching Curt about strokes, and how to recover from them, it was inevitable that Ron would talk about the new thrust of his work and his passion for looking at diet as the source of non-communicable diseases such as atherosclerosis. Curt also embraced that view and, very quickly, saw that no matter how great the scientific understanding might be, individuals would have to choose to implement the findings in their lives. That meant that his work in Cognitive Behavioral Therapy could be quite relevant. The collaboration was cemented.

Why was it necessary for Ron and Curt to get together to write this book? Let's make that clear. It was because Ron discovered that it was one thing to learn metabolic pathways that support development of atherosclerosis; it was another thing to convince people (patients) to eat appropriately in order to mitigate or avoid atherosclerosis. Since eating appropriately refers to controlling sugar intake, Curt immediately recognized that addiction might be at play in eating habits; at a minimum Curt thought that habituation could be a factor. This fed into Curt's interest in addictions. But, sugar addiction? Not many addictions professionals believed back then that sugar could become addictive.

If the reader doesn't believe that addiction exists, then he or she should try to abruptly stop eating simple sugars such as fructose and glucose. Or, since alcohol also plays a role in the development of atherosclerosis, he/she should also try abruptly stopping alcohol consumption. Of course, everyone knows that alcohol is addictive and, importantly, that it is potentially both an acute and a chronic toxin. We have only fairly recently recognized also that fructose is a chronic toxin that contributes to development of atherosclerosis. It does not matter that fructose is not inebriating. At the very least, it is habituating simply because it tastes sweeter even than glucose. Ron and Curt realized that, as in the case of alcohol, more and more fructose is required to give the same effect. As we take in more and more fructose all of the consequences of obesity accelerate markedly.

Along the way in our collaboration we have added friends and colleagues who have helped us a great deal. One outstanding friend is Elisha R. Injeti, Ph.D., Associate Professor and Director of Research and Development at Cedarville University in Cedarville, OH. A second new outstanding friend is Rocco Rotello, Ph.D., Associate Professor of Pharmaceutical Sciences at Cedarville University in Cedarville, OH. These two fellows have been of tremendous help in terms of identifying relevant literature and in reading what has been written by Ron. Doctors Injeti and Rotello both have excellent educational backgrounds that spur them on to make things better for us humans through their current positions.

So, there you have our story and an explanation of our backgrounds and the passions that have more or less consumed us in recent years. We very strongly believe that, at this time in our lives, our gut feelings reflect known, but cutting edge, science. We know what to do to mitigate atherosclerosis and so will you as you proceed through this book. But, knowing as we do that any health profession educational program is a bit like 'trying to drink from a fire hose', we have attempted here to keep the book concise and in primer form to help students quickly grasp the factors responsible for developing atherosclerosis. Whether one is a medical, nursing, or pharmacology student this book will be useful and enlightening. Because of its primer form, this book will also prove helpful to practicing professionals who are already established in their career paths, should they not have fully comprehended some of the information to which they were exposed as students. It happened to us and it may have happened to them. After all, atherosclerosis remains the number one cause of medically related deaths and, because of its commonness, it is generally considered to be the natural product of aging. We don't think this is anywhere near the truth.

There is prevention of atherosclerosis and there is hope. Both of these are simpler, physiologically, than might be imagined. But, in the final analysis, the afflicted and the potentially afflicted will need to be as passionate about taking charge of their diet, and their life, as we have become. That is a "scientific statement" also.

In developing this book, we decided that although our goal is the same, i.e., avoiding atherosclerosis, our approaches are different. Ron, the physician, is the principal author of the body of Section 1 which presents a dietary approach based on science and Curt, the psychologist, is the principal author of the body of Section 2 which presents a working psychological scientific approach based on cognitive behavioral therapy. They jointly wrote the foreword, prologue, and epilogue.

Finally, Ron and Curt thank their wives (Cecilia and Jane, respectively) for their help with the manuscript and their tolerance of our being compulsively driven to write this book. We also want to thank Joe Vessell, Ron's great-nephew, for rendering the remarkable drawing in this text that relates the configuration of the portal vein.

Glossary

ERFYH   – eat right for your height

T2DM   – type 2 diabetes mellitus

NCD   – non-communicable diseases,
      meaning non-infectious diseases

SAD   – Standard American Diet

GI   – gastrointestinal tract

HFCS   – high fructose corn syrup, a man-made product

VLDL   – very low density lipoprotein,
      the precursor of LDL

LDL   – low density lipoprotein, once oxidized,
      the "bad" cholesterol

HDL   – high density lipoprotein, the "good" cholesterol

mg/dl   – milligrams per deciliter

BP   – blood pressure, mmHg

O2   – oxygen, inhaled via the lungs

ROS   – reactive oxygen species, cause oxidation
      of proteins and fatty acids

DNL   – *de novo lipogenesis*, the making of new fat

TRIG   – triglyceride, three fatty acids bundled
      together on a glycerol molecule

CHOL   – cholesterol

PL   – phospholipids

SREBP-1c   – sterol regulatory element binding
      protein-1c, gene transcription factor
      that works to provoke DNL

ChREBP   – carbohydrate response element binding
      protein, gene transcription factor that
      works to provoke DNL

ACL — adenosine tri-phosphate citrate lyase, enzyme that initiates fatty acid formation in DNL

ACC-1 — acetyl-CoA carboxylase-1, enzyme that prepares citrate for conversion to fatty acids

FAS — fatty acid synthase, enzyme that synthesizes palmitic acid from precursors in DNL

ELOVL-6 — elongation of very long chain fatty acids-6, enzyme that elongates fatty acids formed in DNL

SCD-1 — stearoyl-CoA desaturase-1, desaturates saturated fatty acids

GLUT — glucose transporters -2, -3, and -4, for specific cells, GLUT-5 transporter for fructose

ATP — adenosine tri-phosphate, main cellular energy source for the body

CO2 — carbon dioxide, gas excreted via the lungs

Krebs Cycle — citric acid cycle or tricarboxylic acid cycle, performs oxidative metabolism in mitochondria

NAFLD — non-alcoholic fatty liver disease

NASH — non-alcoholic steatohepatitis, inflammation of the fatty liver

LPL — lipoprotein lipase, gate keeper enzyme that frees fatty acids for transfer into bodily cells

NEFA — non-esterified fatty acids, bound to albumin in bloodstream

JNK-1 — c-jun N-terminal kinase 1, an enzyme that blocks proper activation of insulin receptors in the liver

HSL	– hormone sensitive lipase, enzyme that frees intracellular fatty acids from triglycerides
BMI	– body mass index, kg/m²
BMDAC	– bone marrow derived angiogenic cells
•NO	– nitric oxide free radical (the "•" denotes a free radical whether O_2 or NO)
CHO	– carbohydrate
FAT	– fat
PROT	– protein
NCEP	– National Cholesterol Education Program
US	– ultrasound, a process used to assess for atherosclerosis of arteries
EBCT	– electron beam computed tomography, used to assess coronary arteries
CPK	– creatine phosphokinase, enzyme that reveals muscle destruction
calories	– we use the small "c" for calories as a convention for kilo-calories usually spelled with a large C
AA	– Alcoholics Anonymous
CBT	– cognitive behavioral therapy

Prologue

*F*or the past several years, the authors have been reviewing research papers and texts on basic lipid chemistry and cognitive behavioral studies regarding eating habits, along with pouring over news clips and magazine articles trying to glean information regarding our national health crisis. We did this to justify a proper dietary approach, after concluding that we Americans are, to say the least, a medical mess. Two-thirds of us are overweight or obese with many heading toward atherosclerotic disease or developing or have already developed type 2 diabetes mellitus (T2DM) often without knowing one is doing so/has done so. The same is happening now to our adolescents and teenagers. It doesn't mean that the slender are immune to this collective metabolic tragedy, otherwise known as the non-communicable disease (NCD) epidemic of medicine. While the slender are far less likely to develop T2DM, this is not necessarily so where developing atherosclerotic (athero… Greek for porridge-like material, sclerotic…Greek for hard) plaques in one's arteries is concerned. In fact, the metabolic tragedy of NCD's we are experiencing is overwhelming the population with atherosclerotic disease or hardening of the arteries. Atherosclerotic disease is principally what leads to heart attacks, strokes, ruptured aneurysms, and peripheral vascular disease and the need for vascular surgery, inclusive of heart and kidney transplants. It is often complicated by two major lipid disorders, fatty liver disease and excessive fat deposition in the muscle cells of one's extremities and heart. Moreover, there is a long list of additional ailments that accompany consumption of the Standard American Diet (SAD), a term now used by Michael Pollan the food guru.[1] Among these (not listed in any particular order) are cancer (colon, prostate, pancreas, liver, kidney, esophagus and breast), chronic kidney disease, kidney stones, gastroesophageal reflux disease, sleep apnea, diverticulosis of the colon, erectile dysfunction, dementia (vascular and possibly Alzheimer's disease as well), osteoarthritis, gout and dental caries, to name a few.

Who is to blame? Well, let us start with agribusiness and the processed food industries. We are being served things that are not real food or if real, food that is often contaminated directly or indirectly with antibiotics, hormones and bacteria. One cannot expect, for example, to eat meat derived from corn-fed beef cattle maintained in totally crowded feces-adorned feed lots without eventually meeting up with a bad bacterium such as *Escherichia coli* or to eat eggs from fowl or the flesh of fowl raised in similar conditions without fear of an occasional exposure to *Salmonella typhi*, the latter being the prime bacterial cause of infectious gastroenteritis. Several strains of both of these two bacterial organisms, *E. coli* and *S. typhi*, can cause illness severe enough to result in death. Some strains of *S. typhi* are now known to be antibiotic resistant. This probably reflects use of antibiotics by the growers particularly of beef, pork and fowl. More recently, we have been hit by a scourge of *Listeria monocytogenese* bacterial infections linked to cantaloupes, of all things, which potentially underscores this organism's presence in the GI tracts of ostensibly healthy people who work the fields. A number of people have died due to the *L. monocyteogenes* episode. These problems are pretty obvious and they immediately suggest hygienic issues in our food chain, as they well should.

What is not so obvious is what is happening with processed foods. By processed, we mean anything baked, cooked, canned, bottled or otherwise concocted outside of one's home to prolong shelf life. There is an interminable list of such foods. Clever chemists and nutritional scientists have learned how to manipulate the three sirens of the processed food industry (salt, fat and sugar) to play on the taste buds and habitual behavior of individuals. To these, they add a list of ingredients, including odors, which can also provide mechanisms for impacting habitual behavior. A simple loaf of bread, e.g., may have in addition to glucose derived from the starch of wheat, sucrose and high fructose corn syrup (HFCS) and an additional list of ingredients often of somewhat specious need but also sometimes behavioral in action but sometimes helpful such as iodide. Why? We don't know about all the other ingredients but we do know something about the three sirens, more specifically about the carbohydrate (CHO) or sugar siren. Let us not forget that people in the processed food business are there to make money. What they serve up has no bearing on whether or not it is healthful; the bearing is on whether or not the food is bought often and is profitable in the market place.

In the aforementioned trio, our focus is primarily on CHO's, specifically the simple sugars fructose and glucose and alcohol. Though you won't find drinkable alcohol in processed foods very often (it evaporates on cooking), it is a commodity that is clearly and obviously readily available otherwise. Fructose and glucose are most often applied to processed foods as sucrose (table sugar from beets or cane, a 50%-50% mix of the two sugars) or as HFCS, (usually 42-55% fructose to 58-45% glucose mix, the most common mix being 55% fructose and 45% glucose, where fructose is enzymatically derived from the glucose of corn starch) or regular corn syrup (100% glucose derived from corn starch). Believe it or not, all three are sometimes applied in the same processed food: read the ingredient labels. Even more sugar is sometimes added in a very concentrated form known as fructose syrup (about 90% fructose).

We follow the metabolism of these CHO's and how they abet the development of body fat and, accordingly, how they play into the scheme resulting in atherosclerosis. We have developed a dietary approach that obviates the need for eating a plant-based diet (the vegan approach) to improve vascular health. The elegant work by Caldwell Esselstyn, M.D. of the Cleveland Clinic shows that a plant-based diet devoid of meat, fish, eggs, poultry, dairy, nuts, certain vegetables, vegetable oils and fat sprays is heart healthy. He has observed that a diet devoid of fat (FAT) and cholesterol (CHOL) can improve atherosclerotic lesions of one's coronary arteries, even reverse such lesions. While not stressed by Esselstyn, a vegan diet often brings with it weight loss, meaning that the tendency to imbibe energy in excess of need is reduced.[2] This is certainly a healthful aspect of such a diet.

We feel that the vegan approach would prove a hard sell to most Americans and perhaps to others around the world and, if utilized exclusively, it would be too disruptive of our agrarian economy. It is also apparent that such a restrictive approach is not needed unless, e.g., one has advanced kidney disease but, in this circumstance, a vegan diet is more likely to be used for reasons other than mitigation of atherosclerosis. At the end of this text, we provide an epilogue on how to deal with our health crisis. It may not be appealing or liked by all, perhaps by very few, for a variety of reasons but it will surely work and it will help provide less toxic food for those of poor or modest means who experience more obesity, diabetes and atherosclerotic disease than most.

And, finally, let us deal with one other aspect of the American healthcare system. On a piece-work (read incentive) basis, it has been devoted almost entirely to treating the end result of eating habits, not in developing a preventive approach to our long list of NCD problems. Be assured that drug manufacturers, medical device manufacturers, specialized physicians, hospitals, insurers and others are quite attuned to this long list of problems. Collectively, over the years, these groups have made trillions of dollars off of our inability as a nation to address the primary cause of our NCD problems. Our efforts at treating the end results of NCD's are impressive but are also very, very expensive. Such efforts may prove helpful in the short haul, even prolong life, but, on the whole, they solve none of the problems because they do not get at their root cause. This is why Medicare and Medicaid are becoming unaffordable as we now know them and why, in fact, private health insurance is becoming prohibitively expensive for many. It is why all forms of health insurance are likely to become unavailable in the long term unless we introduce preventive measures. It is time to address the issue of health care from a common sense dietary strategy, one quite likely acceptable to the masses and one that can be supported at both federal and state levels. Be aware that billions have been spent on drug discovery research programs targeting obesity but most all drugs have essentially failed or proven toxic in their own right. No one, no country, no government can afford to treat what is happening; it is a "bank buster" of the first order. Highlighting this prior statement, a recent magazine article summarized the magnitude of our healthcare problem in dollars, $2.6 trillion in 2010 to be specific. The article noted that we in the U.S. spend more on health care than France does on everything (housing, food, healthcare, education, defense, infra-structure, etc.) making the U.S healthcare debacle the fifth largest economy in the world in terms of dollars spent.[3]

Summary

De novo lipogenesis (DNL), the making of FAT in the liver, results in the production of very low density lipoprotein (VLDL). The production of VLDL represents a bodily mechanism for balancing nutrients internally to provide control over energy stores and blood glucose levels. Much more FAT can be readily stored than can glucose, a factor visually apparent in our U.S. population. VLDL, in fact, is the liver's main export module for certain nutrients. VLDL carries fatty acids in their triglyceride (TRIG) form, phospholipids (PL) and cholesterol (CHOL) to all bodily cells. Due to distribution of its nutrient contents, VLDL becomes low density lipoprotein (LDL) and, once oxidized, the so-called "bad" CHOL. Moreover, VLDL production is much more responsive to CHO intake than to FAT intake. LDL additionally provides nutrients to our cells but it also becomes, once oxidized, a prime causative factor in atherosclerosis, a disorder principally involving one's larger arteries of distribution. The biological management of LDL exhibits a "systems-biology weakness". This occurs because of the high oxygen (O_2) content in one's arterial blood and the significant blood pressure (BP) in one's larger arteries. Excessive CHO intake, which provokes DNL in the liver, drives the availability of LDL but also directly leads to blood-borne and, presumably, subendothelial glycation of LDL's protein (PROT) rod and oxidation of both its PROT core and lipid contents. Glycation occurs in the high O_2 atmosphere of arterial blood and causes oxidation of the LDL particles through the production of reactive oxygen species (ROS). Movement of both intact and oxidized LDL particles through the interstitial or intercellular spaces of the one cell layer thick endothelial linings of one's larger arteries to the subendothelial area is enhanced by the significant BP.

Deposition of subendothelial atheromata (Greek…plural of atheroma) comprised of oxidized LDL leads to activation of one's innate immune system which attempts to digest and clear the atheromata or plaque material within one's larger arteries but which does so ineffectively when there is a profusion of oxidized LDL particles. In time, arteries so affected dilate and also experience dense calcium deposition due to ongoing inflammation surrounding the plaque material. A vulnerable atheromatous plaque may rupture into the arterial lumen to cause vascular occlusion or, far less commonly, outwardly to cause a hemorrhage. Two other lipid disorders, excessive *ectopic lipogenesis* within the liver and within the striated muscle cells of one's heart and extremities, often occur concomitantly with atherosclerosis, particularly in the overweight and obese. Such problems may worsen atherosclerosis because of global involvement of the innate immune system in all three conditions. From a logic viewpoint, excessive production of VLDL is a link to all three disorders.

We conclude that the optimal treatment of atherosclerosis is dietary, in conjunction with statin therapy, if needed. Reduction of CHO intake, through minimizing fructose, moderating glucose and moderating or avoiding alcohol consumption, is key to reducing oxidized LDL to levels manageable by the innate immune system. All three disorders, i.e., excessive *ectopic lipogenesis* within liver and muscle cells and atherosclerosis, respond to reduction of inflammation through proper diet and weight loss, if the latter is needed. If weight loss is not needed, only change of the macronutrient composition of one's diet is required. Because of the insidious nature of atherosclerosis, often followed by a vascular apocalypse in middle age, if not before, it is recommended that treatment to target lipid levels be instituted years before middle age arrives with diet first or with diet plus a statin, if indicated. Recognizing that there are behavioral aspects surrounding sugar consumption, we have also provided a working program to help reverse the addiction to sugars. It is based on cognitive behavioral therapy but parallels the "step process" used by Alcoholics Anonymous (see Section 2).

Avoiding Atherosclerosis

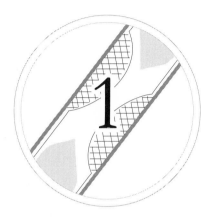

Section One
A Scientific Approach to Diet

1.1 Introduction

Cardiovascular disease due to atherosclerosis remains the number one medical cause of mortality in the U.S. and worldwide because of heart attacks, strokes, ruptured aneurysms, and peripheral vascular disease. Cardiovascular disease has been noted to cause 38% of all medically related deaths in North America and is the most common cause of death in European men under age 65 and the second most common cause in adult European women.[4] To provide further insight on prevalence of atherosclerosis, it has been reported that there are 1,350,000 acute coronary syndromes annually in the U.S.[5] But, often over looked clinically are the lipid disorders frequently associated with cardiovascular disease, namely, excessive *ectopic lipogenesis*, i.e., deposition of fat within the liver cells and the muscle cells of one's extremities and heart.

There are probably several ways the above three disorders can interact but principal among them is the innate immune system, a system that evolved over eons to ward off microbial invaders to preserve the host on a reflexive acute basis, not a chronic basis. When turned on continually to cause chronic inflammation, as is the case in atherosclerosis, the innate immune system can provoke harm. This portion of our immune system is involved in atherosclerosis partly because of the presence of pathogen-like molecules (e.g., phosphorylcholine present in some bacteria as well as in oxidized LDL CHOL.) An in-depth discussion of silent (painless) inflammation and the innate immune system is beyond the scope of this text. However, it should be appreciated that studies have shown that hypercholesterolemia can cause focal activation of innate immune activity, reminiscent of delayed hypersensitivity, beneath the endothelium of large and medium size arteries. There is up-regulation of vascular-cell adhesion molecule-1 (VCAM-1) receptors on the luminal side of endothelial cells. Circulating cells such as monocytes and T-cell lymphocytes of one's adaptive immune system carry counter-receptors and adhere to the endothelial cell surface through the VCAM-1 receptor and are then attracted to the subendothelial area.[4] All cells attracted to the endothelium enter (squeeze through by *diapedesis*—Greek, for walking through) into the subendothelial area through the interstitial spaces that demarcate cell boundaries.

In essence, based on post-mortem evaluation of arterial plaque material, the breadth of the innate immune system is represented in arterial plaques of humans, including T-cells, macrophages derived from monocytes, mast cells and dendritic cells. The latter three cell lines possess either scavenger or toll-like receptors. The scavenger receptors of macrophages ingest pathogen-like molecules directly and degrade them proteolytically, while the toll-like receptor also binds such molecules but degrades them through a cascade reaction that results in the production of inflammatory cytokines, proteases and cytotoxic oxygen and nitrogen free radical gases.[4] Most likely there is cross-talk between the innate immune system and the autocrine (cell-bound) endocrine system comprised of eicosanoid (long-chain fatty acid) hormones. Such hormones rely on second messengers for intercellular communication. The eicosanoid system is present in all nucleated bodily cells. Operatively speaking, it is best to have ample anti-inflammatory eicosanoids on balance, as opposed to pro-inflammatory eicosanoids. This is the reasoning behind taking supplements of the Omega-3 Oils, eicosapentaenoic acid (EPA) and docosahexaenoic acid (DHA). Omega-3 oils are healthful for essentially all of us, particularly those of us who don't eat cold water fatty fish with great regularity.

We believe the primary intent of the silent inflammatory response in atherosclerosis is to remove the offending agent, i.e., oxidized LDL, its lipid remnants and the cellular detritus deposited from the inflammatory response. However, when overcome by an ongoing excessive burden of oxidized LDL, the inflammatory aspect becomes an issue in and of itself. The presence of smoldering inflammation can lead to plaque disruption, causing a spillage of its contents either into the arterial lumen to cause occlusion of blood flow or extravascular through rupture of an aneurysm to cause a hemorrhage. How vigorously and appropriately the innate immune system is balanced is important. There is evidence in mice that supports a role for tonic control of the innate immune response via two anti-inflammatory cytokines, interleukin 10 and transforming growth factor β.[4]

The foregoing discussion may explain why some people with relatively high levels of LDL CHOL do not develop aggressive atherosclerosis (high anti-inflammatory response) while, in contradistinction, some with normal, even nominally low, LDL CHOL levels express aggressive atherosclerosis (high pro-inflammatory response). Supporting this variability in response, of course, is one's underlying genetic structure obligate to avoiding or developing atherosclerosis. Gaussian distribution is at play in such medical problems. Implicit in the message, here, is that "what and how much one eats and how often" influences immensely the innate immune and the autocrine hormonal systems and the balance of the "good" and "bad" in each system. The reader's personal study of inflammation involved in atherosclerosis is certainly warranted and encouraged.

Silent inflammation may exist for years before the apocalypse occurs and the pain arises due to either atherosclerosis or the often associated excessive *ectopic lipogenesis* within liver cells and muscle cells of one's heart and extremities. The coupling of the latter two nonvascular lipid disorders with the vascular lipid disorder may provide a reason as to why atherosclerosis often advances more aggressively in overweight, obese and diabetic individuals. Being overweight or obese additionally serves to aggravate the vascular inflammation because of the presence of inflammatory cells attracted to the FAT cells of the greater omentum within the abdomen and the array of cytokines and other chemical factors they produce and release into the circulation. It is important to remember that we are all different biologically to some extent; it is those at risk whom we seek out to protect. In the case of atherosclerosis and the often associated disorders due to *ectopic* deposition of fat, the "at risk" group comprises a huge segment of the U.S. population.

It is imperative that we be able to additionally explain cardiovascular deaths that occur not only in those with excessive body weight but also in those of apparently normal body weight. To do so, one might consider sudden death in distance runners such as those that occurred in the 2009 Detroit Marathon (three men in their mid twenties to mid-fifties dropped dead during the marathon). [an interactive web site for runners (http://www.runnersworld.com)] In addition, a 40 yo female had a heart attack and may have survived and a 64 yo male died during the swim portion of the New York Triathlon in August, 2011.[6] Another contender died of a heart attack in the 2011 Louisville Triathlon.[7] More recently, two men dropped dead at the end of the November 2011 Philadelphia Marathon.[8] There is also the interesting story of a 54 yo male Cincinnati runner who fell in an unconscious state toward the end of the 2010 Thanksgiving Day 10k Race. He was resuscitated at the site and moved quickly to a hospital where he promptly underwent 4-vessel coronary artery by-pass surgery. He apparently swore to run again in the 2011 Cincinnati 10k Race, though we could not confirm that he did so. The Cincinnati runner serves as a prime example of cardiac arrest due to coronary artery disease. He had been a runner most of his life.[9] Although the actual cause of death is unknown to us in the majority of cases (autopsy information is not always available), death among marathon, triathlon and 10K runners seems to be an ever present, if not growing, problem. Because of the growing popularity of such sporting events, such deaths tend to illustrate the specter of latent cardiovascular disease.

Two recent articles highlight the concern over sudden death in distance runners. The first article deals with the nature of the cardiac problems. Many affected runners, as would be expected, had developed exercise-induced *hypertrophic cardiomyopathy* and electrical conduction problems but some also had coronary artery disease, with or without *hypertrophic cardiomyopathy*. Such issues predominate in men more so than in women. Of the 59 cases of cardiac arrest reported in this paper, 42 were fatal.[10] The second article details findings in three male marathoners, ages 45, 55, and 49, who either developed chest pain, first two runners listed, or became unconscious, the 3rd runner listed, immediately after completing the 2011 Boston Marathon. All three men experienced "exercised-induced" atherosclerotic plaque rupture and arterial occlusion. All were saved through immediate medical attention at the scene, followed by prompt coronary angiography and placement of one or more stents to clear and encase the plaque rupture sites. The fellow who lost consciousness had severe three-vessel disease and, in fact, required three stents in one artery. All three men survived.[11]

We speculate that atherosclerotic related deaths of ostensibly slender and certainly well conditioned distance runners occur because of a dietary "throughput" phenomenon which contributes to coronary artery disease even in those who appear to be the epitome of health. That is, one can stay slender through extreme exercise but produce excessive VLDL that leads to excessive production of oxidized LDL being deposited in his/her coronaries. This is particularly true if one eats or drinks CHO's excessively and experiences the heavy breathing associated with exercise that can inflate even more one's arterial blood oxygen levels for prolonged periods of time. Distance runners are well known for their "carb loading" habits. They do this to enhance glycogen stores in their muscle cells. Their "carb loading" occurs with a combination of both glucose and fructose. "Throughput" is an important concept, one that deserves considerable thought and surely applies even to nonextreme exercising, even nonexercising, slender people.

Electron beam computed tomography (EBCT) scans for screening the coronaries of extreme athletes for calcium deposition may be in order, certainly for older runners, in spite of radiation exposure, expense and the fact that some amount of coronary artery disease can exist without the detectable presence of calcium. However, if calcium is detected, then one can say firmly that atherosclerosis of the coronary arteries is present. The issue then is to determine whether or not this is a medically significant finding. Screening with electrophysiologic studies may also be in order to identify people who might have conduction problems due to exercise-induced *hypertrophic cardiomyopathy*. Medicating older extreme runners with known atherosclerosis with 40-81 mg/d of aspirin (as an anticoagulant factor) along with daily Omega-3 Oils on a chronic basis (as an antichaotic rhythm factor) might be in order. Reducing caffeine intake to none for several days prior to running would probably also help. The training, alone, of such athletes may set them up to have vascular inflammation. Also, running in the morning during cool or cold weather may accentuate the impact of a potent native thrombotic agent, plasminogen activator inhibitor-1, because it is usually at its circadian peak in the morning. One might want to alter his/her time of running to when ambient temperatures are higher.

While reading this section of the book, there are certain thoughts to keep in mind.

• Some amount of imbibed fructose and alcohol is converted to fatty acids in the liver before they are utilized either in oxidative phosphorylation to produce energy in the form of adenosine tri-phosphate (ATP) throughout the body or are stored as FAT in the greater omentum of the abdomen or elsewhere. Glucose, if eaten excessively, can also be converted to fatty acids but at nominal intake levels, it is far less likely to do so in any substantial amounts. In rank order of proclivity to form fat by DNL, we estimate that fructose is first, alcohol is second and glucose is a distant third.

• Coconsumption of excessive amounts of CHO with FAT creates an energy excess state which drives the production of VLDL and, hence, oxidized LDL availability, a prime causative factor of atherosclerosis. It is worth noting that CHO intake triggers DNL, not CHOL intake that everyone focuses on. CHO induced DNL can also utilize fatty acids or TRIG's that comprise the liver's pool of fatty acids.

• Through control over the amount and type of imbibed CHO's, atherosclerosis can probably be mitigated in the vast majority of the U.S. population. There will always be certain genetic disorders in existence (e.g., heterozygous familial hyper-cholesterolemia, incidence 1 in 500 persons, which causes premature atherosclerotic disease due to very high LDL levels because of inadequate LDL receptor sites for clearing LDL) that may require different considerations. Such people along with other types of even rarer genetic problems comprise only a small fraction of the population. Regardless, many people with genetic disorders would probably also benefit from our dietary recommendations.

• Glucose can be imbibed alone when eaten as starch while fructose is typically never imbibed without its companion sugar, glucose. The two together can foster a host of medical problems through interactive mechanisms. This thought is fundamental to developing a prescription for a proper diet.

• It is generally helpful to view, in operative terms, glucose as the "good" sugar and fructose as the "bad" sugar when it comes to lipid production, although at low intake levels, fructose seems to improve glucose production and storage in the liver. Conversely, at very high levels of intake, glucose may be as "bad" as fructose where lipid production is concerned. Fructose (a 5 or 6 member ring structure) is an isomer of glucose (a 6 member ring structure) that is arranged differently in space than glucose. Fructose metabolism differs greatly from that of glucose and, importantly, fructose does not directly stimulate insulin secretion as does glucose.

The discussion in Section 1 deals first with the root cause of the associated lipid disorders and second with the cause and treatment of atherosclerosis. Time is spent on the broader aspects of lipid metabolism so that the reader can develop a more comprehensive appreciation of the interactive aspects of lipid metabolism with atherosclerosis. Focus is on excessive production of VLDL that contributes to fatty liver disease and to excessive *ectopic* deposition of nonoxidized FAT in one's striated muscle cells of the extremities and heart but also on deposition of oxidized LDL in the subendothelial spaces of one's large and medium size arteries. Interestingly, we could find no evidence for excessive *ectopic* deposition of fat in smooth muscle cells present in one's arteries, although the intimal cells are clearly involved in the atherosclerotic process. Once oxidized through blood-borne PROT glycation, due mostly to the sugars and alcohol one eats or drinks, LDL becomes a harbinger of atherosclerosis. Another lipoprotein carrier particle, the chylomicron, the result of DNL in the wall of the small intestine, is also evaluated in its contribution to these three problems.

Before entering into the following discussion on CHO and FAT metabolism, the reader may find it helpful to review a diagram (Pg. 14, Fig. 1, What You Need to Know). This diagram shows the unions of the veins of the intra-abdominal organs to form the portal vein that leads to the liver. Every intra-abdominal organ has a vein that leads to the formation of the portal vein which is pivotal to delivering absorbed nutrients to the liver. The spleen, while not delivering any absorbed nutrients to the liver, is important to recovering iron from senescent red blood cells that are removed from the circulation by the spleen. Such iron has the potential for becoming toxic (via production of ROS) and it is moved quickly to the liver where it is attached to carrier PROT's, such as ferritin, that reduce the potential for iron toxicity. Of course, there are other factors recovered from the spleen, inclusive of B-cell antibodies produced in the spleen that are representative of one's adaptive immune system. The lacteal (micro-lymphatic) system of the small intestine (shown in dark color running like little humps along the small intestine) is not labeled but it is critical to recovering chylomicrons from the *villi* (Latin for hair-like projections) of the small intestine (see 1.15). The chylomicrons reach the bloodstream following the coalescence of the lacteals which contributes to the formation of the thoracic lymph duct that connects to the bloodstream by way of the left subclavian vein.

The diagram also shows the duct leading from the gall bladder to the small intestine that delivers bile acids which assist in the absorption of long-chain fatty acids in the small intestine. The pancreatic duct is shown as well, as it is critical to getting proper digestive enzymes to the chyme (food that has been partially digested in the stomach) within the small intestine and in regulating the pH of the chyme through addition of sodium bicarbonate to neutralize gastric acid. These two ducts merge into the *Ampulla of Vater* and flow into the small intestine from each duct is controlled by the *Ampulla's Sphincter of Oddi*. These two structures are not shown as such in the diagram. The *Ampulla* is only open for drainage into the small intestine during food intake. The gastric or stomach veins are shown prominently. They contribute to the portal vein, as well. It is worth noting, however, that they have branches that extend upward even to the distal end of the esophagus. This early recovery point for glucose, assuming the transporter, GLUT-4, is available in the esophageal mucosal cells, may be particularly important to diabetics who are experiencing a low blood glucose level. This is because some of orally imbibed liquid glucose can by-pass the small intestine and move directly and quickly into the general circulation by passing on through the liver to the hepatic vein. The "fatty apron" (noted as the greater omentum) draped over the transverse colon represents a place where one stores excess fatty acids in the form of TRIG's. The fatty apron has venous drainage directly into the portal vein. It is notable that the colon, portions of which may be retroperitoneal as opposed to intraperitoneal, has venous drainage directly into the portal vein through the superior and inferior mesenteric veins. Many nutrients are recovered at the colonic level, although the colon is generally viewed as a bioreactor that contributes to stool formation because of its high bacterial content.

Finally, it is important to note that the pancreatic vein merges with the portal vein. This allows for much of the insulin produced in response to a glucose load to be adsorbed within the liver to blunt what could otherwise be an excessive surge in arterial blood insulin levels in response to glucose. Much of the insulin produced in response to a glucose load never gets past the liver where it can be bound and biodegraded. Moreover, much of the insulin that does get into arterial circulation is filtered by the kidneys and is further biodegraded in the proximal tubules of the kidneys. This reflects the body's major effort to avoid overload of the arterial circulation with insulin. People with advanced chronic kidney disease due to T2DM often think they are getting better and can lay down their insulin syringes. Unfortunately, they are often shocked to learn that this is not so. They, in fact, are getting worse in terms of kidney disease. Because of advancing kidney disease, they have lost one of the feedback loops for reducing serum insulin levels which, even in situations where pancreatic production of insulin may be on the wane, causes insulin levels to rise and may cause episodes of hypoglycemia. The drainage of the pancreatic vein also permits glucagon, another hormone secreted by the alpha cells of the pancreatic islets, to go directly to the liver to initiate glucose release and production, respectively, through *glycogenolysis* and *gluconeogenesis*. There is essentially a continuous effort to maintain blood glucose levels in a fairly tight range, about 75-90 mg/dl, through the counter action of these two hormones.

All of the foregoing discussion of Figure 1 (see next page) illustrates how important and central the liver is to the management of imbibed nutrients. What is critical, once this well orchestrated arrangement is appreciated, is to understand that it can be either friend or foe, depending upon what, how much and how often one puts food in his/her mouth.

Figure 1: "What You Need to Know"

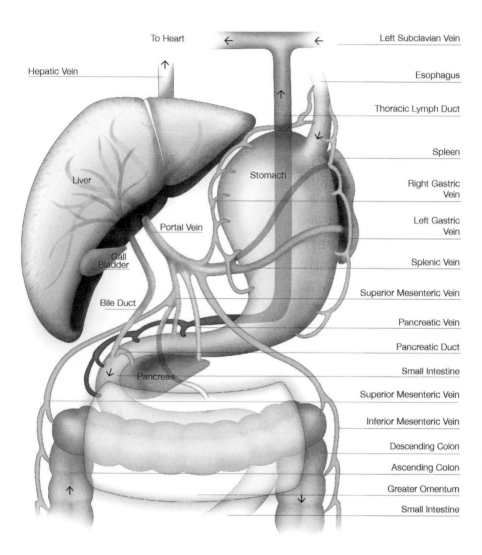

To Heart

Hepatic Vein

Left Subclavian Vein

Esophagus

Thoracic Lymph Duct

Spleen

Liver

Stomach

Right Gastric Vein

Left Gastric Vein

Portal Vein

Gall Bladder

Splenic Vein

Bile Duct

Superior Mesenteric Vein

Pancreatic Vein

Pancreatic Duct

Small Intestine

Pancreas

Superior Mesenteric Vein

Inferior Mesenteric Vein

Descending Colon

Ascending Colon

Greater Omentum

Small Intestine

1.2 Synthesis of VLDL

The human liver has the ability to synthesize VLDL containing TRIG's consisting of fatty acids from either the existing fatty acid pool within the liver or the fatty acids derived from certain imbibed CHO's and, probably to a far lesser extent, directly from imbibed short- and medium-chain fatty acids and their TRIG's. The process, regardless of the origin of the fatty acids, is referred to as DNL which, in the case of CHO's, includes their conversion to fatty acids as well as their conversion to their FAT or TRIG form by means of esterification of fatty acids with a glycerol molecule followed by attachment of the TRIG's to the Apolipoprotein B100 (Apo B100) PROT rod of VLDL. Coincidentally, this PROT rod is one of the longest PROT's known to exist in humans. The esterification process occurs as follows: TRIG's, whether arising from existing fatty acids or newly synthesized fatty acids derived from CHO, are made by attaching 3 fatty acid molecules sequentially to each of the 3 alcohol moieties of a 3-carbon glycerol molecule. A water molecule is formed at each esterification point. Synthesized TRIG's, regardless of the origin of their fatty acids, cannot be stored safely in the liver to any major extent. They are principally incorporated into VLDL particles along with two other lipid groups, PL's and CHOL, and exported from the liver into the general circulation. As indicated earlier, VLDL is the liver's main export module for conveying these factors into the general circulation within one's body.[12] The DNL process results from the activation of gene transcription factors which enter the liver cell nucleus, directly or indirectly, to activate genes that result in the production of enzymes that lead to the formation of VLDL. Although the VLDL level is often present on one's lipid report, the report does not differentiate as to the origin of the fatty acids of VLDL. But, if VLDL levels are elevated, one can be almost certain that CHO intake is excessive relative to need.

The gene transcription factors required for sugar conversion to fatty acids are now established. Fructose, while perhaps less well documented than glucose, appears along with glucose to have the ability to activate both CHO response element binding protein (ChREBP) and sterol regulatory element binding protein-1c (SREBP-1c), to provide the essential transcription factors required to initiate DNL of fructose and glucose. Fructose activates ChREBP through the enzyme protein phosphatase 2a, stimulated by an intermediate of fructose metabolism, xylulose-5-P, and activates SREBP-1c through stimulation of peroxisome proliferator-activated receptor–Υ coactivator-1β by fructose-1-P produced in the initial glycolytic step involving fructose.[13] Glucose activates ChREBP by controlling its entry into the cell nucleus and by activating the binding of this transcription factor to one's DNA. Glucose also stimulates insulin secretion and insulin activates SREBP-1c which, in turn, acts through a nuclear receptor known as LXR-α to activate genes within the cell nucleus.[12] So, alone or together, fructose and glucose can activate the two transcription factors that activate genes within the liver cell nucleus to encode the production of all enzymes required to generate fatty acids up to 18 carbons in length. Such enzymes reside in the cytosol of liver cells and include: adenosine tri-phosphate citrate lyase (ACL), acetyl-CoA carboxylase-1 (ACC-1), fatty acid synthase (FAS), elongation of very long chain fatty acids-6 (ELOVL-6), and stearoyl-CoA desaturase-1 (SCD-1).[12] We have assumed, but have not found this to be completely defined in the literature, that the three CHO's of interest in this text are all subject to the actions of these five enzymes. In the case of alcohol, it may be that FAS is the terminal enzyme so that only the saturated fatty acid, palmitic acid, is produced. Regardless, all three CHO's provoke DNL.

1.3 Management of fructose

When eaten, fructose is absorbed in the jejunum of the small intestine by means of the sugar transporter GLUT-5 oriented toward the liver in the enterocytes of the small intestine. This allows fructose to flow directly to the liver in the portal vein. Once fructose reaches the liver cells, GLUT-5 transporters also assist entry of fructose into the liver cells.[13] This is a very efficient process and little fructose escapes the liver. Because of the glucose that always accompanies the fructose in one's CHO food sources and the frequent consumption of the complex CHO known as starch, which is comprised entirely of glucose molecules, only a minor portion of imbibed fructose is normally converted to lactate. Lactate can be utilized by bodily cells, including the brain, as an energy source. However, conversion of fructose to lactate in the liver is generally suppressed by an increase in insulin secretion secondary to the concomitant intake of glucose. Insulin's action causes carbon from fructose to remain in the glycolytic pathway to form pyruvate which can then enter into oxidative phosphorylation in one's mitochondria in the liver, once transformed into citrate.[14]

Fructose, which is not imbibed without its dietary partner, glucose (except experimentally), does not in either of its isomeric forms stimulate insulin secretion. The beta cells of the pancreas do not express the transporter, GLUT-5, at any significant level. However, as has very recently been found, fructose can potentiate the effect of glucose on insulin secretion by the beta cells as demonstrated by *in vitro* studies. It does so through "taste bud like" sensor proteins present in the pancreatic beta cells which secrete insulin. Studies have been performed on both human and mouse pancreatic islets. The importance of this finding in regard to lipid metabolism in the human remains to be established.[15] All initial metabolism of fructose occurs only in the liver. Most fructose that escapes the liver either recirculates to it to continue the action of inducing VLDL production or it is excreted in urine. The tiny microfilters of the kidneys (the glomeruli) off-filter fructose from the water in one's blood plasma into the urine. However, unlike glucose, there is no transporter mechanism for its absorption back into the body's circulation. Indeed, in the human, urinary excretion of fructose can be used to estimate sucrose or table sugar consumption, this being a 50-50 mixture of fructose and glucose.[16] In the case of glucose, there are sodium-glucose cotransporters present in the cells of the microtubules of the kidneys and these effectively reabsorb glucose from filtered urine nearly to extinction in individuals with normal plasma glucose levels and normal kidney function.

Fructose does contribute somewhat to the production of glucose via increased *gluconeogenesis* (the making of new glucose) due to the 3-carbon moieties resulting from its unique glycolytic pathway, as evidenced by small increases in blood glucose levels after fructose administration. Once in glycolyisis, however, fructose metabolism by-passes a key enzyme, phosphofructokinase, which allows one of fructose's main intermediary metabolites, glyceraldehyde-3-P, to be shunted directly into making pyruvate and, hence, citrate which gives rise to fatty acids via DNL.[17] Thus, fructose is principally cleaved into two 3-carbon compounds which can be turned into pyruvate in glycolysis that is used to synthesize citrate for oxidation within the mitochondria in the Krebs Cycle to generate ATP, CO_2 and water within liver cells. Fatty acids are synthesized in the cytosol after excess citrate leaves the mitochondria by a mechanism known as the "citrate shuttle." There is no true regulatory impediment, here, as there is for glucose. In effect, the more fructose one eats, the more FAT one produces. The "citrate shuttle" comes into play because mitochondrial oxidative metabolism is a rate limited process. An excessive burden of fructose to make citrate prompts action of the "citrate shuttle." It is unlikely that the low level of fructose in fruit turns on the "citrate shuttle;" this is because most people do not eat more than one apple or orange or a handful of grapes at a sitting. Moreover, the fiber of fruit slows the absorption of their sugar content which further aids in avoiding the turn on of the "citrate shuttle" in the liver.

The liver is at risk for experiencing the effects of ROS during metabolism of fructose which is essentially totally focused in the liver until it is transformed into TRIG's. This is because during glycolysis an aldehyde, glyceraldehyde-3-P, and a ketone, dihydroxyacetone-P, are produced. The aldehyde can potentially provoke ROS formation that is damaging to liver cells through PROT glycation. Dihydroxyacetone-P can be converted to glyceraldehyde-3-P via an isomerase enzyme to further glyceraldehyde-3-P production and the ROS problem.

Excessive DNL to form fatty acids in the cytosol of liver cells, whether due to fructose, glucose or alcohol intake, slows mitochondrial beta-oxidation of fatty acids that produces energy because of the build-up in malonyl-CoA required to make fatty acids in the cytosol. This build-up inhibits carnitine palmitoyl transferase-1, an enzyme that regenerates carnitine from the carnitine-fatty acid complex that shuttles fatty acids into the mitochondria from the cytosol for oxidative phosphorylation.

This inhibitory process leads to some accumulation of fatty acids within the cytosol of liver cells.[12] Some of this build-up is offset by their utilization to form TRIG's that are attached to the B100 PROT rod, a process stimulated by CHO induced DNL.

1.4 Management of glucose

Glucose, when consumed in moderation, has a far, far lesser direct impact on DNL, compared to either fructose or alcohol, partly because it is subject to the rate limiting enzyme phosphofructokinase in glycolysis.[17] Importantly, glucose is utilized readily in the liver to make glycogen (the storage form of glucose as a starch) or as is true for most glucose consumed, it can be utilized directly by all nucleated bodily cells to produce ATP by means of oxidative phosphorylation within cellular mitochondria, once it passes through glycolysis. Liver glycogen, unlike muscle glycogen, can release glucose to be used throughout the body. This is because muscle cells do not contain an enzyme to remove phosphorous from glucose-6-phosphate. Since most glucose moves on through the liver into the general circulation or is packed into glycogen within the liver, this, in essence, dilutes its ROS impact on any single organ or tissue or cell. Once in glycolysis in any cell, it produces the same two chemical forms produced during the glycolysis of fructose, glyceraldehyde-3-P and dihydroxyacetone-P, to increase the risk for developing ROS. The ROS potential of glucose is distributed and thereby diluted, as indicated, among one's trillions of nonliver bodily cells so that should ROS arise, they can be quenched more reliably by antioxidants to avoid cellular damage.

When glucose is eaten in moderation and is absorbed and enters the portal vein under the influence of its transporter GLUT-4 in the jejunum, about one-fifth transfers into liver cells through the action of another glucose transporter, GLUT-2, to form glycogen to meet later glucose related energy needs. The balance of about four-fifths of glucose intake flows directly on to all bodily cells, particularly those of the cerebral cortices of the brain whose cells possess the insulin independent glucose transporter, GLUT-3, to contribute to the oxidative production of one's chief molecular energy source, ATP, in the brain.

Very little glucose, when taken in moderate quantities, perhaps even in fairly large quantities depending on energy balance of the individual in question at any given time, is converted to the mono-unsaturated fatty acids, palmitoleic and oleic acids, as discussed later (see 1.7). Regardless, glucose derived from excess starch, lactose and maltose consumption, not from just sucrose and HFCS, must be considered in the balance that could lead to enhanced fractional DNL and the "lipid droplet" problem in the liver, as discussed later (see 1.11). It is worth noting that substantial amounts of glycogen, a watery starch, can be made and stored in the liver without any ill effects.

The production of VLDL, primarily stimulated by fructose since its initial metabolism is focused in the liver, reveals the fact that the mitochondria within liver cells have limited capacity for oxidizing citrate in the Krebs Cycle to ATP, CO_2 and water. This is a rate dependent catabolic process modified by one's thyroid status, exercise activity and altitude and cold exposure.[18] When this rate limitation is exceeded through excess inflow of pyruvate (clearly in the case of even moderate fructose intake and minimally in the case of moderate, perhaps even large, glucose intake) into liver mitochondria to form citrate, the "citrate shuttle" in liver cells is called into action, this feature being provided by the mitochondrial transporter family.[19] As indicated earlier, citrate then moves out of the oxidative pathway present in mitochondria into the cytosol of liver cells to produce acetyl-CoA that contains the 2-carbon foundation used in the synthesis of fatty acids and CHOL. The conversion to acetyl-CoA occurs via the action of the enzyme, ACL. The enzyme ACC-1 then converts acetyl-CoA to malonyl-CoA which is used by the enzyme FAS to form palmitic acid, as discussed further below (see 1.7).

1.5 Annual consumption of sugar

The primary interest of this discussion is neither the starch present in grains and vegetables nor the fructose and glucose present in fruits, berries, honey, maple syrup and molasses, although the latter three sources could clearly cause health problems if consumed excessively. All three approach both industrially produced sucrose or table sugar and HFCS in terms of their fructose and glucose contents. Rather, the primary interest, here, is in sucrose and HFCS which, by far, account for the two major and nearly equivalent industrial sources of fructose and glucose in the so called SAD. Most processed foods contain such sugars and the household use of sucrose and HFCS abounds, as well. It has been reported that, from the beginning of the 20th Century to the present, the *per capita* intake of fructose has increased by a factor of about five. The 2010 Disappearance Data tracked by the USDA indicate that Americans, per individual, now annually imbibe about 156 lbs of sugar or 0.4 lbs/day or 182 gm/day (about 50% fructose and 50% glucose) when the sucrose, fructose and glucose (all three are present in most fruits) from fruit drink intake is added to the disappearance data. This represents a doubling of fructose intake over the past 30 years or so. In contrast, FAT intake has remained relatively stable over the same time-frame.[13]

1.6 Management of alcohol

Alcohol, i.e., ethanol (a 2-carbon moiety with a hydroxyl group attached), enters the portal vein directly by diffusion (it is highly soluble in water) and then the liver cells by diffusion from the portal bloodstream, after a small amount is absorbed and metabolized in the cells lining the stomach and small intestine. Once in a liver cell, alcohol is converted to its aldehyde form, acetaldehyde, by the enzyme alcohol dehydrogenase-1B. The aldehyde can also glycate a free amino group of a PROT and cause production of a ROS and through propagation of the ROS, unless terminated by an antioxidant, oxidize both FAT and PROT within the liver cells. Logic suggests acetaldehyde probably has at the most an intermediate impact of the three CHO's on blood-borne PROT glycation (fructose first, alcohol second and glucose third) but, of course, this depends on the amount consumed of any of the three CHO's, singularly or simultaneously, and whether or not blood glucose levels are elevated by the presence of diabetes. Acetaldehyde, even in the absence of glucose intake to stimulate insulin secretion, can directly activate the gene transcription factor, SREBP-1c, to initiate DNL. This appears to be the only gene transcription factor utilized for DNL from alcohol in the absence of sugar intake. The aldehyde is then converted to acetic acid by the enzyme aldehyde dehydrogenase-2. Acetic acid is then buffered to form sodium acetate. Acetyl-CoA synthetase, an enzyme present in the cytosol of liver cells and also a SREBP-1c target gene, can achieve production of acetyl-CoA which provides the foundation for making either fatty acids in the DNL process or CHOL. From this point on, the same enzymes are operative that are used to make fatty acids from fructose or glucose, at least up through the utilization of the enzyme, FAS, but possibly also through all five enzymes to create fatty acids up to 18 carbons in length. Fatty acids derived from alcohol can attach to the Apo-B100 PROT rod of VLDL as TRIG's.

There are two other pathways that can be utilized to metabolize alcohol in the liver and elsewhere of far lesser quantitative significance. One is the microsomal ethanol oxidizing system. This is a pathway induced in the liver in individuals who consume alcohol chronically. The other pathway is a non-oxidative pathway catalyzed by fatty acid ethyl ester synthase which results in the formation of fatty acids in both the liver and the pancreas. This pathway is thought to provide substantial oxidative stress in the liver and pancreas because of lipotoxicity. [20]

A standard serving size for alcoholic spirits is about 1.5 oz or 43 gm. Alcohol is viewed as having about 7 Atwater calories per gram. In the standard serving size of 80 proof spirits (40% alcohol by volume), the caloric value is rounded off to around 100 calories, a value that coincidentally takes into account some of the energy cost (diet induced thermogenesis) related to the metabolism of alcohol. However, when viewing the caloric input from standard serving sizes for wine (about 5 oz) and beer (about 12 oz), one has to subtract any associated Atwater calories (4 cal/gm) of glucose or fructose to reveal the caloric impact of alcohol, itself. Again, the Atwater caloric values do not take into account any energy cost of their metabolism. Fructose probably has a somewhat greater cost due to diet induced thermogenesis than glucose because so much of the former is converted to FAT for the production of VLDL. Glucose, on the other hand, is primarily oxidized directly in the Krebs Cycle of cells throughout the body to produce energy. And, finally, one has to consider the possibility that in light alcohol intake versus heavy alcohol intake, alcohol may be managed differently in metabolism. That is, light alcohol intake might favor sodium acetate production while heavy alcohol intake might favor FAT production. We could find no evidence that this possibility has been examined in laboratory experiments but it is a consideration.

It is worth noting that metabolism of alcohol evolved not to metabolize the alcohol of spirits, wine and beer but to metabolize the several types of alcohols normally present in some food sources (e.g., berries); these are typically not the kinds of alcohol that cause inebriation or liver or brain damage. As spoken to later (see 1.10), much of the alcohol one consumes in a modest single dose is converted to sodium acetate within the liver. Sodium acetate can evade being turned into acetylCoA in liver cells by moving freely into the bloodstream for dispersal to all bodily cells. Once inside of nonliver cells, it is converted to citrate, following which it is metabolized oxidatively in the Krebs Cycle of the mitochondria to the exclusion of fatty acids.

1.7 Fatty acid conversion products of DNL

The conversion of fructose, glucose, and alcohol to the long-chain saturated fatty acid, palmitic acid, occurs in the DNL process. Palmitic acid, 16-carbons in length, then, in the case of glucose and fructose (and probably alcohol), either remains in its native form or it is desaturated to form palmitoleic acid, a mono-unsaturated fatty acid, by SCD-1. Or, it is further elongated by means of the enzyme ELOVL-6 to form an 18-carbon stearic acid molecule which is then desaturated by SCD-1 to form the mono-unsaturated fatty acid, oleic acid. The TRIG's of fatty acids, principally those of the mono-unsaturated fatty acids, are attached to the Apo B100 PROT rod to form VLDL through the action of microsomal triglyceride transfer protein. Two additional lipid groups, PL and CHOL, as indicated earlier, are added to the Apo B100 PROT rod. [12] It should be noted that TRIG's containing palmitic acid have been identified in the blood of humans at substantial levels rather promptly after fructose intake, as DNL turns on rather quickly.[21] TRIG's are a major source of energy when stored in FAT or muscle cells or when transported in the bloodstream to other bodily cells. The unsaturation of some of the palmitic acid residues reduces what otherwise would be an overwhelming burden of a 16-carbon saturated fatty acid. When *steatosis* of the liver (fatty liver disease) occurs, however, such fat principally contains the TRIG's of oleic acid.[12]

1.8 TRIG's *of fatty acids*

The TRIG's derived from the liver's fatty acid pool that can also be contained in VLDL particles could be comprised of (in terms of probability) virtually any fatty acid available, irrespective of chain length or degree of saturation. The liver pool contains fatty acids that either have just been eaten and flow directly to the liver from the small intestine (short- and medium-chain fatty acids or their TRIG's) or have been recirculated to the liver from peripheral depots such as abdominal FAT cells and the muscle cells of one's extremities and heart (typically long-chain fatty acids). Another type of lipoprotein carrier particle, the chylomicron, originates in the small intestine to accommodate dispersal in one's body only of long-chain fatty acids just eaten. Such fatty acids may recirculate to the liver's pool of fatty acids, as well. Moreover, some of the fatty acids recirculating to the liver were initially a part of previously produced VLDL and, thus, face reincarnation as VLDL for re-export into the bloodstream. If VLDL is made up only from fatty acids derived from CHO or from fatty acids initially attached to chylomicrons, all such TRIG's of VLDL will be comprised of long-chain fatty acids. More is said below (see 1.15) about chylomicrons and their own separate intestinal DNL process.

VLDL particle diameter or size varies mostly because of differences in TRIG content per VLDL particle but somewhat because of the wide range of fatty acid sizes in the liver's pool of fatty acids and also because TRIG's of saturated fatty acids pack more tightly in the VLDL particle than do TRIG's of unsaturated fatty acids. Once in the bloodstream, such particles can further vary in size because their component parts are continually being removed for cellular energy purposes (fatty acids) or cell structural or product synthesis purposes (fatty acids, CHOL and PL). And, there is particle remodeling that goes on rather continually through the action of other enzymes and particles which can adjust VLDL particle size upward or downward, both within the liver and within the bloodstream. A nominal range of widths for VLDL particles is 30-80 nanometers, where 1 nm = 1 billionth of a meter. The three major passenger constituents of VLDL are: TRIG (55-80%), PL (10-20%) and CHOL (5-15%). [22]

1.9 Negative physiologic impacts of alcohol and fructose

For alcohol, we have no figures estimating consumption but, based on availability, we assume it is prodigious in spite of being costly and heavily taxed. It is best to avoid or limit its consumption because, among other reasons, it is metabolized to form VLDL via DNL in the liver to, thereby, create LDL particles that cause atherosclerosis while simultaneously depositing "lipid droplets" in liver cells, as spoken to later (see 1.11). Alcohol can also adversely affect one's brain cells because of its aldehyde form, acetaldehyde, which causes inebriation due to its anesthetic action on nerve cells. Acetaldehyde also creates ROS through PROT glycation that can induce liver and nerve cell death or *apoptosis* unless promptly quenched by antioxidants. Since fructose is also changed to FAT via DNL in the liver, it is reasonable to deduce that either fructose or alcohol, alone or together, can cause fatty liver disease and, alone or together, ultimately cirrhosis of the liver. This is due mainly, we think, to the focused production of ROS in the liver derived from fructose and alcohol that denature PROT and FAT through oxidation which results in scarring and collagen deposition; a cirrhotic liver is truly a scarred organ. In either case, the cirrhotic liver no longer contains FAT because of the death of its (formerly) metabolically active cells, the hepatocytes. Various approaches have been attempted to inhibit or reverse liver cell death through caspase and caspase-independent pathways by IDUN Pharmaceuticals, now part of Pfizer. Fortunately, fructose, while it may have scant presence of its GLUT-5 transporters in various hedonic or mesolimbic pathways of the brain, is not metabolized in the brain directly for energy nor does it cause inebriation nor can it cross the blood-brain barrier of the cerebral cortices due to the absence of its transporter, GLUT-5, in the endothelium of the cortical vessels.

Both fructose and alcohol qualify physiologically as chronic toxins, though only alcohol is viewed by society as being both an acute and a chronic toxin. The ability to minimize fructose intake today is very difficult because of obfuscation in food labeling and the preferred use by the food processing industry of solutions that contain fructose and glucose in the form of either sucrose or HFCS or both, sometimes jointly with corn syrup which contains only glucose and also sometimes jointly with fructose syrup which is nearly pure fructose. The corn processing industry has recently sought permission to refer to foods or drinks with HFCS in them as containing "corn sugars" to further complicate understanding what's in a food. Fortunately, the FDA refused to allow relabeling as "corn sugars." Shelf life of processed foods is prolonged because bacteria cannot readily utilize fructose in its sugar form to generate energy and because of the fact that food processors remove most fiber from the initial food product to further improve shelf life. Removal of fiber reduces the water content of processed foods which limits bacterial mobility and bacterial commune development, i.e., food processing limits the production of bacterial biofilm. It is worth remembering that human mitochondria cannot metabolize fructose until it has been transformed into either glucose, lactate, citrate or fatty acids, all being products of metabolism in the liver. The food processing industry recognizes that fructose is also more habituating (if not addicting) than glucose because it tastes sweeter. In short, we have no need for federal or other agencies or groups to promote fructose (e.g., the USDA and the corn-soybean-wheat, agribusiness, food processing and chain restaurant lobbies). We do have need, however, for federal agencies to control fructose consumption (such control might rest with either the Health and Human Services Department, the Bureau of Alcohol, Tobacco, Firearms and Explosives, the Center for Disease Control and Prevention or the Food and Drug Administration) to protect our nation's people.

There are a number of physiologic ways that fructose declares it is a toxic substance in humans when eaten repetitively at high dose levels. But, since its adverse effects are not precipitous and all are chronic in nature, fructose toxicity is ignored by both the food industry and the US government (including the presidency and congress, and the FDA, USDA, and CDC) to the detriment of society. We suspect that policy decisions at the federal level will be required to eliminate fructose presence in processed foods and drinks. It will be an uphill battle for a variety of reasons. Policy mandates are the only way to manage major public health problems such as those brought on by excess fructose intake.

1.10 Concept of fractional DNL

It is clear from the literature that, in the human, there is a direct relationship of fractional DNL in the liver attributable to CHO intake and that variation in total DNL in the liver is related much more to CHO intake than to direct FAT intake. In fact, FAT consumption has very little direct impact on VLDL production via DNL. Excessive CHO intake (whether fructose, glucose in large amounts or alcohol), on the other hand, can drive the DNL process and worsen health issues. The DNL involving the liver's fatty acid pool probably continues 24 hrs/day to some extent in all humans because fatty acids are continually being exported back into the bloodstream and recirculated to the liver in some amount from one's other bodily cells, particularly from muscle cells and abdominal FAT cells contained in the greater omentum. This organ has venous drainage (by means of the superior mesenteric vein) directly into the portal vein that leads to the liver. The transfer of free fatty acids from FAT cells and muscle cells into the bloodstream is also a problem that worsens with being overweight or obese, certainly in those who are either insulin resistant or diabetic. This is because energy intake exceeds energy need in such people, due mainly to excessive consumption of CHO with FAT.

The DNL derived from the liver's fatty acid pool may exceed CHO driven DNL on the whole, as the latter occurs only intermittently with food intake throughout the day with respect to total VLDL production in the liver. Of course, this makes a key point: The amount of fractional DNL clearly depends upon how much fructose, glucose and alcohol one consumes each day and, perhaps, on how often they are consumed. There is strong evidence which suggests that DNL from CHO sources, particularly fructose, represents an induction process.[21] Thus, the amount of fructose, for example, that one imbibes with breakfast may influence how readily the liver metabolizes the additional influx of fructose for conversion to fatty acids with the intake of food thereafter each day. Alcohol definitely turns on fractional DNL. In one study, fractional DNL before challenge was 1% but after a 24 gram bolus challenge of alcohol, it rose to 31%.[23] The fractional DNL attributable to 24 grams of alcohol is a little misleading in that only about 5% of the single dose of alcohol in this study was converted to fat. Most is converted to sodium acetate in the liver, as indicated earlier, which then diffuses into the bloodstream to supplant fatty acid oxidation in cellular mitochondria throughout the body through formation of citrate. This slows oxidation of fatty acids in the mitochondria and may contribute to some of the hypertriglyceridemia seen after heavy alcohol consumption. The paper just cited did not look at multiple serial hits with alcohol, so we are not sure if the same pattern prevails with heavy drinking. If alcohol intake is heavy enough, the "citrate shuttle" is turned on to further lipid production in the cytosol of liver cells. Fructose and glucose, if the latter is eaten excessively, and alcohol induce fractional DNL and, in doing so, may prepare the liver for additional doses of each or all three throughout the day.

Fractional DNL from CHO observed in lean people on a high FAT diet has been noted to be a little less than 3% of total DNL.[24] However, in obese insulin resistant people, where CHO energy intake principally from simple sugars and starch exceeds energy need, the fractional DNL rose to greater than 10%.[25] Radiotracer studies in obese people with known *steatosis* of the liver (fatty liver disease) exhibited greater than 26% fractional DNL.[26] In other studies on people consuming a high CHO diet, DNL rose by a factor of 27 in the fasting state versus fasting DNL when on a low CHO diet and by a factor of 4 in the fed state versus DNL when on a low CHO diet.[27] In still another human study, a comparison of fractional DNL was 2% versus 10% with equivalent dosing after 6 days of either a high glucose or high fructose intake, respectively.[28] This latter finding rather clearly underscores the use of glucose to make glycogen and to be used directly in oxidative metabolism, as opposed to being principally converted to fat in the liver as is true for fructose.

Since the concept of fractional DNL may be a little esoteric, we analyzed a very comprehensive review article[29] that quotes numerous research papers which show that moderate to high fructose intake, whether as sucrose or fructose, alone, is almost invariably associated with *post-prandial* hypertriglyceridemia, the majority of such TRIG being carried by VLDL. Prolonged exposure to fructose can also cause an increase in fasting total CHOL and LDL CHOL in the majority of studies but not in all. This indicates that fasting total CHOL, TRIG and LDL CHOL, as would be predicted, are probably more limited indicators of the effect of fructose on DNL since some people clear TRIG's and LDL faster than others. *Post-prandial* elevations in VLDL and LDL, however, equals time spent in a potentially atherogenic state due to high VLDL levels giving rise to high LDL levels. Unfortunately, this is something little appreciated in the real world of clinical medicine, mostly because it is both inconvenient and expensive to study patients who are not fasting. What was also obvious in the studies quoted is that glucose intake in the absence of fructose has very little effect on either *post-prandial* TRIG or fasting TRIG levels. In fact, glucose loading seems typically to be associated with both lower than baseline *post-prandial* and fasting TRIG levels. This implies, firstly, that glucose is principally utilized in nonlipid pathways, such as forming glycogen and oxidative metabolism, and, secondly, that the TRIG reducing action due to insulin released in response to glucose (insulin mobilizes the enzyme, lipoprotein lipase as spoken to later, see 1.12) blunts even further any detectable impact of glucose on *post-prandial* or fasting lipid metabolism.

Several studies quoted in this paper also showed that the hyperlipidemia following fructose intake was greater (in one study, dose-dependent) in people with either insulin resistance or diabetes. This may be another reason why such metabolic conditions are associated with greater risk due to atherosclerosis. Several papers in this review suggest, for reasons uncertain, that premenopausal normal weight women are generally less reactive to fructose in terms of its hyperlipidemic action. Post-menopausal women, on the other hand, are more likely to react to fructose feeding in a manner comparable to men, as are overweight women regardless of their menopause status. It is important to appreciate that, in some people, fructose creates a dyslipidemia pattern (low HDL CHOL, high TRIG, and high LDL CHOL) characteristic of the metabolic syndrome.

1.11 "Lipid droplet" problem

TRIG's of fatty acids, once produced via DNL, whether from fructose, glucose or alcohol, are corralled into tiny droplets of fat (a fraction of a micron in size) surrounded by a single layer of either amphipathic PL or CHOL molecules in the cytosol of liver cells. It is unclear to us whether the "lipid droplet" is a feature of DNL occurring prior to attachment of TRIG's to the B100 PROT rod or the result of TRIG's being produced in excess of what will fit onto the B100 PROT rod or both.[30a] Regardless, droplet production is linked to TRIG production and the droplet configuration may reduce the potential for fatty acid toxicity (lipotoxicity) because the TRIG's are contained. Such droplets, however, can fuse and grow larger through a complex series of droplet interactions. If energy intake is excessive, it may conceivably drive the process of droplet fusion though some amount of fusion appears to be ongoing independent of energy balance. The "lipid droplet" issue is present even with moderate intakes of fructose and alcohol, whereas with moderate glucose intake, it is probably of minimal, if any, importance both in terms of size and growth. "Lipid droplets" exist in a variety of fluid or tissues besides the liver, such as in breast milk, brown and white fat cells, and striated muscle cells.

"Lipid droplets," while visible only with electron microscopy of biopsy material in the beginning in liver cells, can fuse to become large enough (over a time frame perhaps of years, depending upon eating and drinking habits) to be detectable by US or CT scans to provide the noninvasive diagnosis of *microsteatosis* of the liver or fatty liver disease. The "lipid droplets" are the prime contributor to the development of *steatosis* of the liver; excessive growth in droplet size must be avoided in the human through curtailment principally of CHO intake. "Lipid droplets" in the liver represent a functional form of *ectopic* FAT deposition in an organ central and fundamentally crucial to lipid metabolism. Excessive recirculation of fatty acids and TRIG's in the bloodstream to the liver in overweight, obese, insulin resistant, and diabetic individuals also contributes to the problem of "lipid droplet" growth. Again, CHO intake must be restricted to avoid suffusion of the liver with fatty acids and TRIG's that enhance growth of the "lipid droplets." Doing so allows mobilization and use eventually of a droplet's TRIG/fatty acid content perhaps in DNL or oxidative metabolism by liver cells or other bodily cells after such lipid makes its way into the bloodstream.

Fatty liver disease is often described as a "two-hit" phenomenon, the "first hit" being deposition of fat in the liver (*steatosis*) and the "second hit" being conversion to an inflammatory state (*steatohepatitis* or fatty inflammation).[31] We speculate that the latter occurs due, in part, to the fragility and rupture of excessively enlarged "lipid droplets", whereupon freed TRIG's of fatty acids expose the hepatocytes to lipotoxicity that can cause inflammation and attract cells of the innate immune system to the liver. Moreover, fatty tissue of the greater omentum bustles with immune cells and cytokine products of the innate immune system. These can move freely to the liver by means of the portal vein and add to or perhaps cause the problem of *steatohepatitis*.

The general prevalence in U.S. adults of nonalcoholic fatty liver disease (NAFLD) is estimated to be between 14% and 24%[12], though some estimate that up to 30% of adults have NAFLD.[31] The overall prevalence of metabolic syndrome in the U.S. adult population, where hypertension, obesity, dyslipidemia, gout, insulin resistance and diabetes are major issues, is about 34%.[32] However, this publication indicates that the prevalence of metabolic syndrome grows to about 53% in those with nonalcoholic *steatosis* of the liver (a reversible problem). Metabolic syndrome then grows to a prevalence of 88% in those who exhibit nonalcoholic *steatohepatitis* (NASH) or fatty inflammation of the liver (a very difficult problem to reverse). About 5% of people with *steatosis* of the liver will go on to develop NASH. Of those with NASH, about 25% go on to develop cirrhosis of the liver over time (an irreversible and ultimately fatal disorder). NAFLD is now the most common cause of cirrhosis of the liver worldwide, not alcohol. Clearly, NAFLD is furthered by the presence of being overweight, obese, insulin resistant or diabetic, all being situations where energy intake is excessive relative to need and where fatty acids and TRIG's abound in blood recirculating to the liver to compound the "lipid droplet" issue. Parallel findings, though the numbers are not yet quite as harrowing, now accompany the emerging obesity epidemic in the U.S. childhood and adolescent populations.

1.12 *Impact of glucose on insulin and insulin on* FAT

Importantly, once in the bloodstream during and following a meal, glucose stimulates the secretion of insulin which, in turn, facilitates glucose transport into certain bodily cells. But, once present in increased amounts in the bloodstream, insulin also stimulates the activity of extracellular lipase enzymes. In particular, it stimulates the action of lipoprotein lipase (LPL), the so called "gate keeper" of FAT storage in FAT cells of the greater omentum and in the muscle cells of the extremities and heart. The action of LPL is referred to as extracellular *lipolysis*. That is, it frees fatty acids from the TRIG's of VLDL exported from the liver for diffusion either directly into endothelial cells lining one's vascular system or indirectly into cells within the walls of one's blood vessels through the interstitial or intercellular spaces of the endothelial linings of arteries and veins. But, predominantly, in terms of total mass balance, fatty acids flow through the interstitial spaces of the endothelium in one's vast capillary beds by diffusion to serve the many additional trillions of bodily cells. VLDL also unloads PL and CHOL for nonenergy cellular uses.

In spite of insulin's excessive presence, such as when insulin resistance prevails, its suppressive impact on intracellular *lipolysis* within abdominal fat cells in the overweight and obese becomes muted, as discussed later (see 1.14). Thus, some export of fatty acids into the portal vein from the fat cells of the greater omentum can continually occur by virtue of the fact that intracellular *lipolysis* in fat cells exceeds intracellular *lipogenesis* by some amount. Moreover, if energy intake continues to exceed energy consumption through oxidative metabolism, this provides what is basically a circular process and fat storage continues to increase in spite of intracellular *lipolysis* exceeding intracellular *lipogenesis*. That is, body weight continues to increase. The free or nonesterified fatty acids (NEFA's) emanating from the greater omentum overload the liver and abet the issues of fatty liver disease and oxidative stress. This is because the liver cells respond by taking up fatty acids, irrespective of their concentration in blood flowing through the liver. The foregoing describes the "portal theory of insulin resistance" in the liver. This more extensive form of hepatic insulin resistance occurs well after liver-specific insulin resistance has already been incurred due to the liver's metabolism of fructose, as discussed below (see 1.13).

1.13 *How much* FAT *is enough?*

Once fatty acids are inside one's bodily cells, if not used immediately to meet energy needs via oxidative metabolism, they are normally reconstituted as TRIG's. The intracellular reconversion of fatty acids to TRIG's is called *lipogenesis*. If this occurs in FAT cells for storage, it is referred to as *endopic lipogenesis* and if it occurs in nonFAT cells for storage, *ectopic lipogenesis*. The latter typically occurs in the muscle cells of the extremities and heart but also in and around abdominal organs, especially the liver and elsewhere. Both *endopic* and *ectopic lipogenesis* are normally occurring processes; it is only an issue of how much storage in either case. For example, the required amount of *ectopic lipogenesis* might be viewed as that which provides a "just-in-time inventory" of fatty acids that satisfies the production of one's ongoing need for ATP particularly in muscle cells but also elsewhere. Since ATP is consumed continually to provide energy, the fatty acids need to be provided rather continually, either from fat stores or from fat and sugar consumption at meal time. A normal amount of *endopic lipogenesis*, on the other hand, might be viewed as simply the amount of FAT that provides enough fatty acid storage to meet cellular energy needs in the theoretical but threatening circumstance of starvation for a period of perhaps several weeks, without death as an end result. Trouble arises, however, when storage in both FAT and nonFAT cells prior to starvation can meet energy production needs for several months, even a year or more, in the absence of food intake. This represents a lot of FAT related body weight as is typically observed in the morbidly obese. Such storage can be achieved, however, because of glucose intake that stimulates insulin secretion and excess fructose, glucose and alcohol intakes that are turned into FAT. Because of its propensity to form FAT, one might conclude that fructose is a "FAT masquerading as a sugar," that alcohol is a "FAT masquerading as a CHO," and that glucose, through its stimulation of insulin secretion and insulin's action on LPL, is the "fomenter of obesity."

When both *endopic* and *ectopic lipogenesis* occur in an uncontrolled fashion, FAT storage accrues and health issues arise. This is typified by excess FAT consumption (i.e., the FAT arising from direct dietary intake of FAT and the FAT arising from the intake of fructose and possibly from glucose and from alcohol induced fractional DNL occurring in the liver) and the impact of accompanying glucose consumption that stimulates insulin secretion too often and too much. In this circumstance, insulin drives LPL activity to induce extracellular *lipolysis* to move fatty acids to intracellular locations such as in FAT cells and muscle cells. If the amount of available NEFA's exceeds the storage capacity for TRIG's in FAT cells and muscle cells, then one's bloodstream and tissues become awash in NEFA's which are typically bound to serum albumin for transport in the bloodstream. This is when both *endopic* and *ectopic* cell overload with either TRIG's or fatty acids becomes a major health issue because it leads to a more generalized form of insulin resistance and greater silent inflammation. Thus, generalized insulin resistance supervenes or adds to the initial problem that involved only the liver because of the local inflammatory effects arising from fructose metabolism. Fructose metabolism causes the activation of c-jun N-terminal kinase 1 (JNK-1). The JNK-1 moiety blocks proper phosphorylation of the insulin receptor substrate-1 (IRS-1) in liver cells which causes liver-specific insulin resistance.[13] One way to look at the issue of insulin resistance is to recognize that liver-specific insulin resistance precedes portal hepatic insulin resistance which can precede generalized insulin resistance spoken to next.

Generalized insulin resistance reflects the negative impact of the excess availability of long-chain fatty acids on the ability of glucose to compete successfully in oxidative metabolism in one's bodily cells. Plasma glucose levels rise further due to such insulin resistance and this leads to further increases in plasma insulin levels. And, so on. Insulin resistance does not mean "insulin proof;" insulin's sway over blood glucose to move it into cells still works, just not as well and, similarly, its effect of reducing intracellular hormone sensitive lipase (HSL) enzyme activity continues but less effectively, as spoken to below (see 1.14). Total insulin resistance within one's body is probably the cause of the "sloth" behavior that can accompany obesity; oxidative metabolism just doesn't respond well enough in the presence of insulin resistance. Longstanding insulin resistance, usually after a period of 8-10 years or more, often deteriorates into permanent T2DM.

Over time, as overweightness or obesity develops, insulin becomes less and less effective in facilitating the transport of glucose into bodily cells but it does sustain its ability to stimulate extracellular lipase enzymes to further *ectopic lipogenesis* on top of the excess of NEFA's that are now circulating in one's bloodstream and gaining access to one's tissues and cells. The rising levels of glucose also continue to stimulate ChREBP transcription activity and the corresponding rising levels of insulin continue to stimulate SREBP-1c transcription activity, both being key factors that foster DNL in the liver.[12] It is worth emphasizing again that all fatty acids arising from fractional DNL involving fructose, glucose, if consumed excessively, and alcohol are long-chain fatty acids. Again, the same can be said for the fatty acids of chylomicrons which, by definition, are all also long-chain fatty acids. As insulin resistance advances over time, the perceived cellular need for glucose ultimately calls forth increased secretion of glucagon by the alpha cells of the pancreas that provokes *de novo* glucose release and production in the liver, i.e., *glycogenolysis* and *gluconeogenesis*, for export of glucose into one's circulation. This attempt to meet the perceived need for glucose by bodily cells only complicates the insulin resistance and diabetic issues. This is because, now, there is a major and continuing *endogenous* excess of glucose availability which furthers fractional DNL in the liver 24 hrs/day. This, in turn, furthers the increased availability of long-chain fatty acids via DNL that sustain or worsen insulin resistance. In short, insulin resistance then becomes a closed-loop, upward scaling incremental process. People who present clinically with this problem often require very large amounts of *exogenous* insulin to interrupt *glycogenolysis* and *gluconeogenesis* in order to gain control over blood glucose levels. Such people also often exhibit profound hypertriglyceridemia until blood glucose levels are brought under control. Reduction in CHO related energy intake is a must to gain control over metabolism in such situations.

1.14   *Excessive intracellular lipolysis*

It is important to appreciate that when *endogenous* insulin levels are high, the intracellular HSL enzyme normally becomes far less active, if not inactive. HSL, prevalent in muscle cells, normally responds reciprocally to LPL; i.e., HSL's action is suppressed when insulin levels are high and increased when insulin levels are low. HSL's intracellular action is to free fatty acids from their TRIG configuration for either oxidative metabolism in the cell of origin or for their export into the circulation to meet the oxidative needs of other cells or for storage as TRIG's in FAT cells such as those of the greater omentum. So, from the beginning of the upward spiral in weight gain, if one continues to eat too much glucose too often and stimulates the secretion of insulin too much too often, intracellular *lipogenesis* continues to rise even though intracellular *lipolysis* has also risen because of the failure of the insulin effect on HSL. This contributes to continuing weight gain. Weight loss through reduction in bodily FAT stores, whether in *endopic* or *ectopic* locations, only occurs if intracellular lipolysis exceeds intracellular *lipogenesis* by some amount but, then, only if the resultant NEFA's are consumed in oxidative metabolism, a catabolic process that generates ATP, CO_2 and water. Otherwise, NEFA's and TRIG's are increasingly shifted around in the bloodstream to different sites in the body to no avail. Limiting energy intake in the forms of fructose, glucose and alcohol has to occur to break the cycle. FAT loss from one's abdominal FAT cells and muscle cells of the heart and extremities through weight loss, if overweight or obese, can restore FAT and muscle cell metabolism to a state of normalcy in people formerly exhibiting either insulin resistance or even diabetes.

With adequate weight loss, cell function can recover. For example, the cardiac arrhythmia known as nonvalvular atrial fibrillation, if present, can revert spontaneously to a normal sinus rhythm, if weight loss is substantial. This probably occurs because of reduced inflammation previously imposed by excess FAT storage in cardiac striated muscle cells. FAT or TRIG storage in cardiac muscle cells has been shown to be linearly related to body mass index (BMI = kg/m²).[33] The same can be said for the pancreas; diabetes can be reversed or improved, depending upon the amount of irreversible pancreatic beta cell damage one has already incurred. Clearly, weight loss is a necessity to reverse the reversible forms of NAFLD. Even kidney function, particularly protein loss in the urine, in obese and diabetic individuals can improve to normal with major body weight loss through dietary measures. And, of course, the same measures will aid in reducing the inflammation and progression of atherosclerosis. The key, here, is to reduce energy intake, particularly in the forms of fructose, glucose and alcohol, so that intracellular *lipolysis* exceeds *lipogenesis* in a situation that favors oxidative metabolism of the resultant NEFA's.

1.15 Chylomicrons

Let us turn now to the chylomicrons, mentioned earlier, which are formed in the cells of the small intestine through a DNL process similar to that of the liver but which provides delivery to one's tissues of the TRIG's only of long-chain fatty acids imbibed with each meal. Unlike VLDL that arises from a combination of the liver's pool of fatty acids, the fatty acids of TRIG's carried by chylomicrons are all long-chain fatty acids (14-24 carbons in length), whether poly-unsaturated, mono-unsaturated or saturated. Such fatty acids must be re-arranged in the lumen of the small intestine to form micelles comprised of fatty acids and monoglycerides due to pancreatic lipase that drains into the small intestine through the pancreatic duct. Micelle formation involving bile salts provides emulsification that allows the very hydrophobic long-chain fatty acids we eat to breach the dense mucous barrier of the small intestinal wall to gain access to what are called the *villi* of the small intestine. Each of the *villi* is covered by *microvilli* (microscopic cellular outgrowths) which, collectively, give the small intestinal lining a velvety appearance but which greatly increases the absorptive surface area of the small intestine. Once within the *microvilli*, the fatty acids are rearranged into their TRIG form for attachment to the Apolipoprotein B48 PROT rods of chylomicrons (Apo B48 means 48% of the length of the Apo B100 rod of VLDL). Similar to VLDL, PL and CHOL are also attached to the chylomicron's Apo B48 PROT rod. ApoB48 with its load of nutrients exits the *villi* through the lacteal (microlymphatic) system that merges into the thoracic lymph.

Because of their high TRIG content comprised entirely of long-chain fatty acids, chylomicrons are very, very large fluffy nanoparticles (in median size, about 30-fold greater in diameter than LDL) that gain access to one's bloodstream via the thoracic lymph duct which empties into the left subclavian vein. The chylomicron particles, measuring about 75-1,200 nm in width, unload their cargo to the trillions of bodily cells served by one's vast capillary beds and also to cells lining one's blood vessels. The chylomicron particles have burdens of TRIG 80-95%, PL 3-9% and CHOL 2-7%.[22] They gain access to the walls of one's thicker walled blood vessels, whether arteries or veins, through what is called a *vaso vasorum* (Latin singular for blood vessel feeding a blood vessel), a blood vessel that feeds a capillary bed within the outer smooth muscle or media layer of one's larger arterial vessel walls or the outer walls of thick veins. Specifically, the *vaso vasora* (Latin plural) are blood vessels that feed the outer portion of the walls of blood vessels, whether arteries or veins, with a wall thickness of > 0.5 mm.[34] Though not previously emphasized, here, VLDL and LDL particles similarly gain access to the walls of one's thicker walled arteries and veins. Chylomicrons also unload their fatty acid cargo under the influence of insulin's promotion of lipase activity, along with PL and CHOL.

Remnant chylomicrons, the result of unloading particularly their major cargo of fatty acids but also CHOL and PL in one's tissues, recirculate to the liver where they are digested or cleared by liver cell LDL scavenger receptors, through their interaction with Apo E, another type of lipoprotein. Should any resultant small particles gain access to the circulation and undergo oxidation, then they would also likely be atherogenic or promotional of atherosclerosis. Unlike LDL, however, there is no identified systemic receptor motivated digestive mechanism for chylomicron particles. Our feeling is that they are not atherogenic on any significant scale compared to LDL particles.

1.16 Genesis of "bad" CHOL

Whether derived from DNL involving the existing pool of fatty acids in the liver or from the conversion to fatty acids of imbibed fructose, glucose or alcohol, the VLDL in one's circulation shrinks in size as it unloads its cargo of fatty acids, PL and CHOL. Some VLDL (probably the smaller in size) becomes LDL because of this, while the balance (probably the larger in size) becomes intermediate density lipoprotein (IDL). The IDL recirculates to the liver for further enzymatic reduction to LDL which is then exported back into the general circulation. The three major constituents of LDL are present in far lesser quantities than in VLDL but in inverse proportions to their presence in VLDL (TRIG 5-15%, PL 20-25%, and CHOL 40-50%). LDL nanoparticles measure about 18-25 nm in diameter.[22] LDL, particularly the smaller, denser and more easily oxidized LDL, can readily traverse the interstitial or intercellular spaces of the endothelial linings of all of one's blood vessels which measure about 26 nm in width. The exception, here, is the endothelium of the "blood-brain barrier" protecting the cerebral cortices which has a much tighter porosity (about 1/8 of the porosity, e.g., of the endothelium of arteries and capillaries in one's extremities or elsewhere). The endothelial porosity of the cerebral cortices of the brain, while much tighter, still allows for the passage/transport of NEFA, PL's and CHOL derived from VLDL, LDL and chylomicrons to flow into brain cells through the interstitial spaces due to insulin's effect on lipase enzymes. The brain can exist (after a period of accommodation) on substrates such as lactate and ketone bodies (spoken to below) but favors glucose for energy production over these substrates and fatty acids. Neuronal cells of the brain require fatty acids, PL and CHOL for cell refurbishment and synthesis purposes.

The smaller, denser LDL particles are more atherogenic, i.e., more promotional of atherosclerosis, in one's large and medium size arteries of distribution because they are more easily oxidized by means of PROT glycation, as spoken to below, and probably because they more easily traverse the interstitial spaces that separate endothelial cells. There is some disagreement among lipid scientists about whether all LDL, oxidized or not, contributes to atherogenesis. We have taken the position that only oxidized LDL participates because any nonoxidized LDL would be taken up by endocytosis (as spoken to below) and utilized in metabolism of intimal smooth muscle cells or by other cells beneath the endothelial lining. Oxidized LDL is not capable of undergoing productive metabolism. Oxidized LDL also provokes another issue; it interferes with repair of endothelial cells in vascular walls by bone marrow derived angiogenic cells (BMDAC's). Formerly referred to as endothelial precursor cells, the BMDACs, in fact, are mostly myeloid cells that secrete factors in a paracrine fashion which stimulate endothelial remodeling and which promote vessel stabilization. The BMDAC's do not, themselves, serve to replace damaged or *apoptotic* endothelial cells.[35] Oxidized LDL interferes with the action of the BMDAC's because it reduces the synthesis of nitric oxide, a free radical gas ($\cdot NO^-$), which is one's chief internally produced vasodilator for controlling blood pressure when produced constitutively by nitric oxide synthase in the endothelial cells.[36] There is also an inducible form of this enzyme produced by macrophages within atheromata or arterial plaques which can make $\cdot NO^-$ in potentially harmful amounts. It appears that fructose, as discussed below, and oxidized LDL work in tandem to lower nitric oxide levels either by annihilation of nitric oxide radicals or by depressed synthesis of nitric oxide. Either way, endothelial dysfunction (vasoconstriction) is the result and this leads to increased BP. Such negative effects would be additive regarding repair of damaged endothelial cells.

One of the side effects of ingesting large amounts of fructose is to drive the production of uric acid. This occurs because fructose consumes phosphorous normally recycled to make ATP to, instead, form fructose-1-phosphate in the liver. When this happens, a liver cell's ability to phosphorylate adenosine to form ATP begins to wane. Adenosine, a purine, then shifts, after its phosphorus is scavenged, to the purine pathway that leads to uric acid production. Uric acid is an end metabolite excreted by the kidneys. Excess blood-borne uric acid inhibits nitric oxide synthase in endothelial cells which reduces constitutive •NO⁻ availability. Again, •NO⁻ is one's chief endogenous vasodilator; when availability is reduced, BP rises to further atherosclerosis as a result of endothelial dysfunction. Moreover, we speculate that the circulation of microcrystals of urate is likely very pro-inflammatory in their own right and this may further the subendothelial inflammatory process that causes atherosclerosis even in the absence of clinically obvious gout. The solubility limit for urate in blood, regardless of gender, is about 6.8 mg/dl, at normal body temperature and blood pH. Any level above this can result in crystal formation but not necessarily obvious or classic gout, such as podagra, i.e., pain involving one's big toe.

We would be remiss here if we didn't mention kidney stones as a potential complication of excess fructose intake. This, too, is because of increased production of uric acid which, in acid urine, can crystallize and cause stone formation. Often, uric acid stones serve as a nidus for stone growth through the epitaxial deposition of calcium oxalate. If an apparent calcium oxalate stone is passed, it is necessary to obtain xray diffraction studies of the stone, if at all feasible, to make sure that there is not a uric acid nidus provoking stone formation. The treatment of uric acid stones differs substantially from that of pure calcium oxalate stones.

The apparent nutritional need for LDL is reflected by the fact that each nucleated bodily cell has receptors for LDL, except for those of the cerebral cortices, which allows cells to endocytose the LDL particle in its entirety. Thus, a cell, once LDL is in contact with its receptor (this includes the vascular endothelium of the cerebral cortices but probably not the cortical cells, themselves), invaginates and engulfs the LDL particle to form a vesicle which interacts with other structures in the cytosol that lets the cell gain enzymatic access to its total contents. Endothelial cells that line one's blood vessels can directly endocytose LDL from the blood stream. However, to reach cells within one's larger, thicker walled blood vessels or to gain access to cells contiguous to one's vast capillary beds throughout the body, LDL must move through the interstitial spaces of the vascular endothelium. Once in contact with these more remote cells with LDL receptors, LDL is endocytosed. The endocytosis process is almost assuredly a cell nuclear mediated event, not something attributable to a direct or indirect effect of insulin or any other endocrine hormone. LDL, as explored further below, can become oxidized and form the "bad" CHOL.

It is important to note that there is a rare monogenic defect in producing VLDL and chylomicrons, referred to as abetalipoproteinemia (no Apo B100 and no Apo B48 PROT's are produced, incidence < 1 in 1 million persons). [37] This defect has been known about for years. People so affected can do reasonably well if provided with high doses of fat soluble vitamins, though they tend to die prematurely in their 50's because of progressive neural degenerative problems related to Vitamin E deficiency. Oral mega-doses of such fat soluble vitamins are required to sustain life. Vitamin E, in particular, is normally carried in VLDL. With high dose oral Vitamin E therapy starting early in infancy, progressive neural degenerative problems and retinopathy are markedly attenuated. Patients with abetaliproteinemia respond to diets that minimize long-chain fatty acids but are enriched with short- and medium-chain fatty acids and their TRIG's. This reduces, even eliminates, steatorrhea or diarrhea due to malabsorption of long-chain fatty acids or their TRIG's. In a much more common genetic disorder, heterozygous hypo-betalipoproteinemia (moderate amounts of Apo B PROT's are produced which are somewhat smaller than the normal Apo B48 PROT, incidence 1 in 500 persons).[37] People so affected do well and are long lived, ostensibly because they minimize progressive atherosclerosis. They have total CHOL levels of about 80 mg/dl and LDL levels of about 30 mg/dl and they do not suffer fat soluble vitamin deficiencies due to malabsorption. This genetic disorder strengthens the argument we put forth near the end of this section that the "bar" for LDL blood levels may be set too high for people who can produce lipoproteins normally.

1.17 *How* LDL *causes atherosclerosis*

The impact of LDL is two-fold, one "good" and one "bad". The "good" impact, as discussed above, is to supply nutrients to cells in need either of LDL's contents of fatty acids (energy) or fatty acids, PL's and CHOL (cell refurbishment and product synthesis). The "bad" impact arises, as we relate below, when there is an excess of LDL nanoparticles that become oxidized and are forced through the interstitial spaces of the endothelial linings of the major arteries of distribution by the significant transmural BP and high rotational sheer within one's larger arteries. This places the particles in the subendothelial space and, if oxidized and not amenable to endocytosis and digestion by either the intimal smooth muscle cells or endothelial cells of one's arteries, they are entrapped and provoke inflammation. There is some controversy over whether or not LDL has to be oxidized before it is considered "bad." This may relate to the fact that oxidized CHOL is present normally in one's bloodstream and tissues. However, such normally occurring oxidized CHOL, referred to as oxysterols, occurs in miniscule quantities (as spoken to below, see last paragraph, this chapter) compared to total CHOL or LDL CHOL, and are unlikely, in our opinion, to figure substantively into the cause of atherosclerosis except, perhaps, when specific genetic anomalies exist and an oxysterol might be drastically over produced. We do not know if any such anomalies have been described but it's possible.

Atherosclerosis only occurs in large and medium sized arteries of distribution, not in small arteries or arterioles or capillaries or veins where both BP and O_2 levels become progressively lower. This observation includes the pulmonary artery where BP is quite modest and the O_2 level is at its nadir. Since the subendothelial movement of LDL particles is otherwise occurring in larger arteries in an atmosphere high in O_2 content, there is a greater tendency for the LDL particles to become oxidized within the arterial lumen and presumably beneath the arterial endothelial linings through the impact of ROS. Oxidation of LDL results from an autonomous, nonenzymatic, exothermic process, called PROT glycation, wherein the linear or aldehyde form of fructose or glucose or the aldehyde of alcohol can combine with a free amino group of a PROT. The prime example of this is Hemoglobin A1c which is used to measure the extent of PROT glycation in diabetic patients due to poorly controlled plasma glucose levels (hemoglobin is a PROT within red blood cells that carries O_2 to bodily cells; it's an excellent model of glycation). Each glycation, through release of an electron, produces an O_2 radical which can, if not quenched by an antioxidant, oxidize or denature PROT and other members of the LDL nanoparticle, including CHOL. Such radicals can also annihilate •NO⁻ by adding their extra electron to nitric oxide. The family of ROS free radicals of molecules or ions include: hydrogen peroxide (H_2O_2), superoxide anion (•O⁻$_2$), singlet oxygen (•O⁻), and hydroxyl radical (•OH⁻), in rough ascending order of potency in terms of oxidizing PROT or FAT. ROS are rapidly terminated or quenched by antioxidants such as superoxide dismutase, glutathione and ascorbic acid or Vitamin C, the latter counting among the many, many other antioxidants available through one's diet. Failure to quench a radical leads to oxidative denaturing of PROT that produces scarring or fibrosis from collagen deposition each time a fructose or glucose ring structure unfolds to its aldehyde form or the aldehyde of alcohol is present in the bloodstream to any extent. The combination of significant BP, high O_2 levels and a profusion of oxidized LDL nanoparticles describes the "systems-biology weakness" that has to be remedied in order to mitigate atherosclerosis.

Both fructose and glucose can cause blood-borne glycation of proteins but this event has been shown to occur 7x's more readily with fructose than with glucose through *in vitro* studies. This is probably because one of the former's two ring structures, fructofuranose (5 member ring structure) is not as stable at normal body temperature and blood pH levels as the pyranose (6 member ring structure) noted as follows. The furanose ring structure is common in nature's fruits and berries. HFCS is about a 30:70 mixture of fructofuranose and fructopyranose, respectively. HFCS is made from "field" corn that is naturally very low in fructose content. The production of ROS in the liver from fructose is some 100x's greater[13] than that due to glucose also because fructose metabolism is initially restricted to the liver. Once in glycolysis, it produces glyceraldehyde-3-P and dihydroxyacetone-P as its carbon content moves toward either oxidative metabolism in mitochondria or DNL in the cytosol of hepatocytes. It is important to note, again, that the preliminary metabolism of both fructose and alcohol is largely restricted to the liver. Glucose minimizes its aldehyde form in the liver by conversion to glycogen, a watery starch. Moreover, glucose, but not fructose, is utilized directly in oxidative metabolism throughout the body which, even though it forms glyceraldehyde-3-P and dihydroxyacetone-P in the process, reduces ROS risk through dilution in so many bodily cells. Glucose has only the more stable ring structure in the form of glucopyranose in the blood stream. However, when blood glucose levels rise, as occurs in insulin resistance and in obvious diabetes mellitus, PROT glycation due to an increase in the linear or aldehyde form of glucose also increases. PROT glycation appears to be the primary pathway by which ROS are produced which oxidize LDL in the bloodstream and probably in the subendothelial spaces of one's larger arteries. There is always, always some ongoing PROT glycation in the bloodstream; it is a matter of trying to keep the rate of this process as low as possible. There are, of course, other cell related ways that ROS are produced such as from inadequate mitochondrial oxidation that leads to peroxisomal and microsomal oxidative metabolism of fatty acids in the cytosol of cells. Both of the latter processes are poorly shielded against release of damaging ROS. Moreover, should mitochondrial oxidation become impaired, ROS can result from inadequate membrane respiratory chain management of electrons produced during oxidative metabolism. It should be appreciated that unsaturated fatty acids are more easily oxidized than saturated fatty acids; in fact, there is an exponential increase in oxidation (peroxidation) of fatty acids relative to the degree of unsaturation of carbon-to-carbon bonds.[12]

Macrophages, as discussed below, and endothelial, mast, and dendritic cells all have either or both scavenger and toll-like receptors. The former receptor type takes in oxidized LDL directly and digests it, while the latter receptor type initiates a cascade of events on identifying a pathogen-like molecule that leads to the production of cytotoxic oxygen and, paradoxically, nitrogen radicals both of which assist in the digestion process of the already oxidized LDL particle.[35] While not the subject of this text, excessive ROS production undoubtedly contributes to cancer risk through production of mutations in cellular DNA. The most commonly affected organs were previously listed in the prologue. The reader is encouraged to study the ROS issue and its role, among other things, in cancer.

There have now been identified about 13 molecular species comprised of oxidized cholesterol, more specifically stated, hydroxylated cholesterol. These are referred to as oxysterols; most, but not all, are derived from enzymatic actions involving the P-450 family of enzymes in the liver. A couple of oxysterols result from auto-oxidation like that involving "bad" LDL. Per mole of circulating CHOL, oxysterols measure at the micromolar level. Some oxysterols have been identified in the food we eat. Some correlate with the presence of atherosclerosis and have been identified in plaque material and in sub-fractions of circulating LDL. Oxysterols are typically associated with lipoproteins. They have a broad array of metabolic effects and the liver is the major site of oxysterol clearance. Oxysterols do contribute to bile acid formation in the liver and to bile acid solubility in water and to cholesterol homeostasis. Some are also thought to be anti-atherogenic.[30b]

1.18 *Formation of atheromata*

Once oxidized and deposited within the subendothelial space of an arterial wall, LDL particles form an atheroma (Greek singular for porridge-like material in appearance). An atheroma calls forth action by the innate immune system. Monocytes from the bloodstream are attracted by affected endothelial cells to the subendothelial deposits where they morph into macrophages under the influence of a factor released by the smooth muscle intimal cells of the inner arterial wall.[35] The macrophage cells then engulf and ingest the LDL particles. An atheroma can enlarge in size due to the proliferation of oxidized LDL particles, the accumulation of macrophages and other immune cell lines, including mast and dendritic cells and T-cell lymphocytes and the movement of intimal smooth muscle cells within the arterial wall to more or less encapsulate the atheroma. Once engorged with oxidized LDL, death of the macrophages often occurs, adding to the growing mass. Being an inflammatory process, calcium is attracted and deposits within and around the atheroma. T-cell lymphocytes are called into action for their ability to produce a cascade of cytokines or chemical factors that interact both locally and with more distant cells. Even B-cell lymphocytes from the spleen are involved with atheromata to some extent; they carry antibodies to phosphorylcholine, a pathogen-like molecule common to both oxidized LDL and the cell walls of *Streptococcal pneumoniae* bacteria. People who have had their spleens removed are not only more prone to streptococcal infections but also apparently exhibit more aggressive coronary artery disease.[35]

One of the main problems with the growth in size of atheromatous material and the accumulation of certain enzymes within an atheroma is the potential to cause thinning of the fibrous cap of an atheroma and erosion of the overlying endothelium. Such atheromata are vulnerable to rupture followed by effusion of the essentially foreign oxidized material and cells in the core of an atheroma into the blood stream. If the cap ruptures, platelets, fibrinogen and other thrombotic factors and immune cells are promptly attracted and this can cause interruption of blood flow due to thrombus formation, such as occurs in about 60-70% of acute coronary syndromes.[35] Most atheromata are *ad luminal* in location, but not all. Some are *ab luminal* and can rupture outwardly and lead to a major hemorrhage, such as typically occurs with aneurysms of the cerebral circulation and the aorta. Hemorrhagic events are truly catastrophic and most often lead to sudden death. Fortunately, these occur far less often than the ischemic events. It used to be thought that stenosis of a coronary artery due to atheromatous deposition and luminal build-up of such material was what commonly led to acute coronary syndromes but this appears not to be the case. It is the vulnerable plaques that rupture and are responsible for most acute coronary syndromes. Stenoses represent scarring from accrued atheromatous material and are important to consider, however, as they can cause angina or chest pain because of reduced blood flow through the coronaries. Stenoses are otherwise generally pretty stable lesions. Stenoses can also cause hypertension and even loss of kidney function, if they develop in one or both arteries leading to the kidneys. And, they can also impair blood flow to the brain if present in one or both carotid arteries or larger brain arteries or blood flow to the legs or arms if present in the major arteries feeding the extremities.

1.19 Minimizing atheromata formation

If the number of oxidized LDL nanoparticles is not profuse, the macrophages do their job of removing such debris and move on to other locations; in this case, little calcium is deposited and growth of the atheromata in numbers and dilation of the involved artery is very minimal if at all. This means that atherosclerosis is unlikely to become a killer, at least until one is very old. It is when there is an ongoing profusion of oxidized LDL nanoparticles that atherosclerosis becomes a growth issue, one not tolerable by humans for the long haul. This is because the proliferation of oxidized LDL nanoparticles causes engorgement of macrophages in the subendothelial spaces and the attraction of other immune cells and intimal smooth muscle cells that force the growth of atheromata in numbers and in size and enhance their inflammatory effects which encourages more extensive calcium deposition. The result is often widespread, very dense calcific atherosclerotic vascular disease and arterial dilation that principally affects one's larger arteries of distribution. In this process, thin cap atheromata proliferate as well, increasing the likelihood of either intravascular or extravascular effusion of atheromatous material. This can become clinically apparent in a relatively young age range (e.g., 40-70 years of age) through the occurrence of heart attacks, strokes, ruptured aneurysms, and peripheral vascular disease, if fructose and glucose are eaten excessively or alcohol is drunk excessively or all are consumed excessively, day in, day out. This is true irrespective of an individual's gender or body size, though it worsens with age, particularly if one becomes overweight, obese, insulin resistant, diabetic, or develops chronic kidney disease. Nonoxidized excess LDL recirculates to the liver for complete digestion, if not needed nutritionally.

As indicated earlier, a profusion of LDL particles that become oxidized reflects a "systems-biology weakness" in lipid metabolism. This "weakness" can only be remedied through a major reduction in energy input into one's body, principally in the forms of fructose, glucose and alcohol, an alteration in the macronutrient proportions in one's diet and caloric restriction if one is not at a normal weight for his/her height. Certain pharmaceuticals, such as statins, antihypertensives, antigout medications and aspirin, help reduce health issues resulting from cardiovascular disease but they are far from the final answer in treatment. In this grouping of medications, only the statins have the potential to minimize, even reverse, atherosclerosis if effective in lowering LDL nanoparticle levels adequately. As we speak to later (see 1.21), diet is the most effective means of reducing LDL nanoparticle numbers.

1.20 Reverse CHOL transport

There is reverse transport of CHOL to the liver that may help indirectly to retard growth of atheromatous deposits and growth in atheromata numbers. This is promoted by high density lipoprotein (HDL), the so-called "good" CHOL on one's lipid report. Reverse transport results from an exchange of TRIG's carried by HDL_3 from the liver into the bloodstream with CHOL carried by either VLDL or chylomicron particles present in one's circulating blood to form HDL_2. Following this mutual bilateral hand-off, HDL_2, now with associated CHOL, recirculates to the liver where CHOL is unloaded by an enzymatic process. Some of this CHOL is added to the bile acid pool for excretion from the liver into the small intestine via the gall bladder and its duct leading to the small intestine. This culminates in the so called *enterohepatic* (gut-to-liver) recirculation of bile acids where about 94% are recovered daily and about 6% of bile acids produced are lost daily in one's feces.[38] This repetitive process is related solely to imbibing long-chain fatty acids at meal time. Bile acids are necessary for the emulsification process involving absorption of long-chain fatty acids for attachment to the Apo B48 PROT rod of chylomicrons. Perhaps just as importantly, reverse CHOL transport helps unburden the liver of its TRIG content by providing fatty acids for use elsewhere in the body in oxidative metabolism.

From a clinical perspective, this repetitive bilateral hand-off is why a high HDL level and a low TRIG level on one's lipid report is interpreted as "good" in regard to the nonprogression of atherosclerosis. HDL's small size, 5-12 nm in diameter, allows it to move unfettered in the bloodstream and into and out of extravascular spaces with ease. The high recovery rate of bile acids from the small intestine, on the other hand, suggests that reverse CHOL transport to the liver offers little in the way of controlling VLDL production and the generation of LDL at least at today's levels of sugar and alcohol intakes. This underscores, again, a statement we previously made that reduction in energy intake in the forms of fructose, glucose and alcohol is required for ultimate control of LDL production. This is because VLDL production responds to the intake of CHO, not to the intake of CHOL. HDL can quite likely directly remove oxidized CHOL from atheromata for reverse transport; this has been demonstrated through *in vitro* studies of lipid laden macrophages. HDL also has anti-oxidant and anti-inflammatory capabilities. Evidence also demonstrates that HDL has anti-apoptotic, antithrombotic and anti-infectious qualities toward a broad array of vascular related cell types. These collective actions/properties of HDL may be why multiple observational studies have shown a clear inverse relationship in most human societies between HDL blood levels and the risk of coronary events.[39] The constitutive makeup of HDL is: TRIG 5-10%, PL 20-30% and CHOL 15-25%.[22]

1.21 *Constructing a diet that reduces* LDL *nanoparticle numbers*

We call this dietary approach a method of eating right for your height (ERFYH). From a dietary viewpoint, it is necessary to:

• eat 3 meals daily at appropriately spaced intervals. This will allow one to clear from one's bloodstream the products of CHO ingestion, such as VLDL and LDL, from one meal before the next meal;

• minimize fructose consumption. Eat only fresh or frozen fruits, berries and vegetables, as sources of fructose and glucose to reduce VLDL production and, hence, the quantitative presence of LDL. Avoid fruit and sport drinks, particularly those that have added sugars, and dried fruits because of their high fructose content. It is worth noting that fruit provides one of our main sources of base (alkalinity) to buffer acid incumbent particularly to meat protein, certain dairy products, e.g., cheese, and common table salt. Proper buffering helps minimize the risk of osteoporosis. This is another reason to control salt intake, beyond avoiding fluid retention and high BP. Fruits, berries and vegetables should be eaten with each of three daily meals. If a snack a day is required, it should contain no additional CHO. All desserts should be eaten with meals to avoid an extra insulin spike;

• optimize body weight. One's caloric intake must be correct for one's height, whether male or female. This means that about two-thirds of us need to reduce our caloric intakes. Males generally require about 14 calories per lb of body weight per day, while females generally require about 12 cal per lb of body weight per day. The ideal body weight for the female is 100 lbs for the first 60 inches of height and 5 lbs per inch for anything over 60 inches. For the male, it is 110 lbs for the first 60 inches of height and 5 lbs per inch for anything over 60 inches. For example, if one is a 5'2" female, one's ideal body weight is 110 lbs and the ideal caloric intake is about (110 x 12) or 1,320 calories per day. If one is a 5'8" male, one's ideal body weight is 150 lbs and the ideal caloric intake is about (150 x 14) or 2,100 calories per day. Tables can be constructed that relate caloric intake to each half-inch of height for both females and males covering a span of heights (e.g., 5'0" to 6'6"). The point here, for adults, is that one's height establishes caloric need relative to one's ideal body weight. Ideal body weight relative to height is +/- 10% for differences in body structure, fidget factor, and exercise habits (not including extreme exercise);

• estimate caloric intake per macronutrient using the macronutrient allotment we recommend (35% CHO, 35% FAT and 30% PROT). Multiply the estimated total daily caloric intake by each fractional macronutrient percentage to estimate calories per macronutrient. For total calories to accommodate extreme exercise without weight loss, one may have to use a height that is taller than one is. For example, if one is a 5'8" tall male who runs marathons or is a lumber jack, one may have to plug in a height of 5'10" to 6'0" to achieve a caloric intake that maintains body weight, while keeping the macronutrient divisions spoken to here constant. Daily body weights will keep one informed and allow for adjusting calories and height accordingly; A note about Atwater calories. There will also be some inaccuracy introduced when using the standard Atwater caloric values for PROT, 4 cal/gm, FAT, 9 cal/gm, and CHO, 4 cal/gm. This is because diet induced thermogenesis is not accounted for by the Atwater caloric values. Thermogenesis is greater for PROT than for CHO which is greater than for FAT. In other words, the number of calories one is eating may not be as much as what is advertised. The macronutrient selection we discuss below is higher in PROT intake than most recommended diets but since diet induced thermogenesis is not a great factor in a mixed diet, it is probably of little consequence in terms of losing or maintaining body weight. The macronutrient proportions discussed here are only for adult people with normal kidney function.

• control macronutrient proportions at the levels we recommend (35% CHO, 35% FAT, and 30% PROT). This helps develop satiety when eating because of the PROT and FAT recommendations. The CHO proportion also helps minimize LDL production;

• restrict all fruit and certain vegetable (e.g., potatoes) consumption to meal time. This will avoid an unnecessary insulin response due to the presence of glucose particularly in fruits and berries and certain vegetables. If one must snack, then one should eat something that does not contain significant glucose (e.g., a piece of left over beef, pork, chicken, fish or unsalted nuts);

• moderate or avoid alcohol consumption. This will minimize excess VLDL production in order to further limit LDL level production;

• moderate starch (glucose) consumption. This will avoid additional VLDL and LDL production but also over-stimulation of insulin secretion that leads to excessive *endopic* and *ectopic* deposition of fat derived from either fructose, excess glucose or alcohol. Even though insulin acts as a satiety factor in the mesolimbic area of the brain, this effect can be trumped if too much glucose is eaten. This is because there can be discord between blood insulin levels and blood glucose levels about 2-3 hours after a high glycemic meal. This occurs because the decline in insulin, a peptide hormone (MW 5,808 daltons), is slow relative to glucose (MW 180 daltons) which is quite small and moves rapidly into cells under the influence of insulin. Blood glucose levels can drop rapidly to well below 75 mg/dl. The final determinant over hunger is a low blood glucose level and it is necessary to try and avoid this. Otherwise, one has to eat again, prematurely;

• eat properly chosen nuts that have been a part of the human diet for millennia. If one thinks teleologically, that is, with reason, this is most likely because nuts contain FAT (energy) and some PROT and they are easily stored. There is a ranking available today of Omega-6 Oil to Omega-3 Oil ratio's in nuts. The lower the ratio, the more healthful the nut. Walnuts top the list of healthful nuts;[40]

• optimize PROT intake. Eat meat from grass fed, free range beef and free range pork and fowl and cold water fish and avoid most processed foods. It is healthful to divide total PROT intake into that of meat origin and nonmeat origin on about a 60-40 basis, respectively, to minimize the acid intake incumbent to meat protein. For example, canned black beans, rinsed thoroughly, can serve as a good source of both nonmeat PROT and glucose from their starch. All legumes and lentils provide non-meat PROT and some starch. Rice, quinoa, amaranth, bulgur and barley are similarly good grain PROT sources with only modest amounts of starch. All nonmeat sources of PROT minimize the acid burden otherwise associated with meat PROT;

• control one's metabolism and avoid excessive ketoacidosis. If overweight and attempting to lose weight, adjust caloric intake downward periodically (e.g., every six weeks or so) using fictitious heights until intake is appropriate for one's actual height, using a diet of the proper macronutrient mix. If not overweight relative to height, simple adjustment in the macronutrient mix may be all that is required. Remember, the bathroom scale is the most reliable "calorie counter."

Weigh daily on the same scale, on arising, in the nude. One's goal is to lose no more than 1-2 lbs/wk;

• control inflammation. Minimize consumption of vegetable oils to achieve an improved ratio of Omega-6 oil intake to Omega-3 oil intake. Supplementation with Omega-3 Oils is healthful for anyone. Probably the least vasoactive vegetable oil is Canola Oil derived from rape seeds because of its lower palmitic acid content relative to most other oils.;

• make all of the above changes promptly and simultaneously. Doing so will help restore insulin sensitivity as quickly as is feasible while avoiding excessive ketoacidosis due to weight loss, if the latter is required; and,

• adjust calorie and fluid intakes according to one's height, physical condition, and activity level.

1.22 More discussion on diet

If weight loss is robust in those who need it (i.e., 1-2 lbs/wk but not more), it will not be necessary to make any further adjustment in caloric intake until one hits a plateau that is above one's ideal body weight. Weight loss tells one that fatty acids are being utilized in oxidative metabolism. The shift to fatty acid metabolism is what gives rise to what are known as ketone bodies (acetone, β-hydroxybutyric acid, and acetoacetic acid) during weight loss. If markedly excessive in their presence, they can lower blood pH or increase blood acidity substantially. One's urine can easily be checked for the presence of ketone bodies with a dipstick; if present this tells one right away that his/her metabolism has changed to favor oxidation of fatty acids. The ketone bodies, particularly, acetone, can also alter the odor of one's breath and urine. The main thing to focus on, here, is that fatty acids are being metabolized and are not recirculating profusely to the liver to further either VLDL production and, hence, LDL production or *ectopic lipogenesis* in liver or muscle cells. Weight loss is always accompanied by some amount of ketosis; it's only an issue of how much. Too much ketosis due to excessive reduction in caloric intake, particularly if there is excessive reduction in glucose intake, can cause a major (life-threatening) decrease in blood pH or increase in blood acidity. This can be a problem with the Atkins' Diet, among others. Also, losing weight too rapidly creates hunger and can excessively slow metabolism which makes losing weight more difficult because of the drive to eat. Excessively rapid weight loss can also give rise to gall bladder and kidney stones. Stick with 1-2 lbs/wk, not more. Never, ever "crash" diet.

The problems of excessive *endopic* and *ectopic lipogenesis*, inclusive of fatty liver disease, insulin resistance, and diabetes, is that they are coconspirators in the development and progression of atherosclerosis because of their associated inflammation. All of the foregoing conditions indicate that energy intake in the forms of fructose and glucose and possibly alcohol for many are excessive relative to need. The dietary actions we recommend will collectively improve the age of onset and rate of progression of atherosclerosis and, with dedicated adherence, even reverse several aspects of any existing atherosclerotic disease, particularly if caught early. Such actions will also help reverse fatty liver disease and excessive *ectopic lipogenesis* in muscle cells. As a result, proper dietary measures will increase one's 'health span' within one's theoretical 'life span' of 120 years. Success or failure, where mitigation of atherosclerosis is concerned, is revealed by serial lipid reports, daily body weight measurements and absence of adverse cardiovascular events over time. The critical requirement is to learn how to ERFYH while simultaneously minimizing fructose intake. This dietary approach, coupled with nonextreme exercise, such as brisk walking or biking, can do wonders for one's cardiovascular system (see Section 2, 2.4).

While we recommend macronutrient proportions for adults whose kidney function is normal (CHO 35%; FAT 35%; and PROT 30%), anyone with significant kidney disease will require major alterations in all three macronutrients, particularly in meat PROT intake. As indicated in the prologue, people with advanced kidney disease often have to devolve into eating a carefully orchestrated vegan type of diet in order to survive without requiring dialysis or kidney transplantation prematurely. Carefully orchestrated refers to the need to control serum potassium and phosphorous levels, as well as acid-base balance. The macronutrient arrangement we recommend is categorically a paleolithic diet[40] meant only for people, again, with normal kidney function. Bear in mind that, mathematically, there could be almost a limitless number of combinations of the three macronutrients. The reason we chose the above combination for people with normal kidney function is that the CHO category is low enough to encourage proper fructose restriction while simultaneously discouraging excessive glucose intake and over stimulation of insulin secretion. Providing enough PROT in one's diet also helps avoid consumption of one's own muscle PROT during weight loss to fulfill any need for glucose via the Cori or glucose-alanine cycle, a mechanism for making glucose anew internally from alanine. This amino acid is common to many meat proteins including one's own musculature.

Become an expert in reading food ingredient lists and appreciate that you cannot or should not eat a lot of commercial food products that are available. Sugars are added to many, many processed foods and one doesn't know how much is added (this is considered proprietary information by the manufacturers). One only gets an idea that there may be excess sugar present if it appears early in the ingredient list. If sucrose, HFCS, corn syrup or fructose syrup or all four are listed in the first 5-10 ingredients, return the item to the shelf (remember, the higher on the list, the greater the amount of the ingredient). Of course, there are often many chemicals added with funny names that one doesn't interpret as containing either glucose or fructose but they are sometimes there. To avoid buying baked goods containing excessive sugar, make an apple pie at home with just the sugar (fructose, sucrose and glucose) contributed by the apples. It's delicious and it's low level exposure to fructose. All three forms of sugars are present in most fruits. The crust is just glucose in the form of starch present in flour. The pie should be divided carefully into modest portions and eaten over several days time, not all at once and not as a snack. Eat desserts only with meals, if one has to have a dessert; remember most desserts will stimulate insulin secretion because of the presence of glucose. Finally, one of the most common condiments worldwide today is "ketchup," a tomato product, because of food processing initiated in the U.S. Why don't we figure out a way to make "ketchup" with just glucose but also a variety of spices and herbs that can approximate the allure now due to fructose? Spices and herbs offer almost no calories. If we did this, all BBQ sauces could become healthful over night. And, so on.

If one has abnormal kidney function, one should consult with a kidney disease specialist and dietitian to come up with the proper macronutrient proportions and total caloric intake. This is true because PROT may have to be restricted to minimize acid and phosphate intakes and a build-up in blood urea nitrogen (BUN) levels in one's body and CHO's, specifically fruits, might have to be balanced to avoid excessive potassium intake. Many people have to be changed to a vegan type of diet if their kidney disease is progressive or advanced, in order to avoid premature dialysis or transplantation.

Even with normal kidney function, recognize that there is much controversy surrounding what is an appropriate salt intake. Current recommendations indicate sodium intake should not exceed about 2.0 grams per day or about 5.0 gm of sodium chloride per day. Fluid intake should be commensurate with avoiding lower extremity edema when sitting for prolonged periods. Appropriate fluid intake for shorter adult people with normal kidney function may be as low as 1,000 milliliters (mls) or 2.2 pints per day, while for taller individuals it may be as high as 3,000 mls or 6.6 pints per day or higher. The need for salt and water depends upon urine output, sweat production, and fecal loss of water if diarrhea is an issue. People who exercise and sweat profusely need both salt and water to maintain BP in reasonable limits. It is helpful to remember that a "pint is a pound, the world around," particularly if one has difficulty excreting urine adequately due to chronic kidney disease and is prone to retaining fluid.

All fluids, whether coffee, tea, milk, soda or beer, are essentially water; they just taste differently. Some additional intake in the form of water, only, may be required in certain circumstances. But, in general, ignore advice about drinking eight, 8-ounce glasses of water daily to "flush" one's kidneys in addition to what is drunk in the aforementioned sources of water. Drinking excessive amounts of fluid is nonsense and potentially harmful if it exceeds a rational intake. Salt intake in people with chronic kidney disease must be adjusted to their ability to excrete salt, along with water. Otherwise, fluid retention can become a problem and can result in congestive heart failure. It is probably detrimental, no matter the level of kidney function, to restrict salt excessively because it turns on production of a kidney derived hormone (renin) that can lead to adverse effects such as endothelial dysfunction that paradoxically increases BP which can cause development of punitive cardiovascular issues (as spoken to below). This would certainly prove true in people with advanced atherosclerosis.

Other than when sweating profusely or experiencing kidney stones, fluid and salt requirements are very much related to one's height, as are caloric requirements, albeit the kidneys, if functioning normally, have the ability to conserve salt and water if intake is inadequate or excrete large amounts of salty fluid if intake is excessive relative to need. If one has chronic kidney disease, kidney function will not be so flexible and may be worsened by chronic excessive urine output (e.g., in chronic kidney disease due to adult polycystic kidney disease, an autosomal dominant genetic disorder, excessive fluid output hastens the cystic disease). As kidney function deteriorates, irrespective of cause, the remaining functional units of the kidneys, i.e., the remaining *nephrons*, may be stressed by trying to accommodate an adequate urine output to circumvent excessive fluid retention in order to avoid congestive heart failure. Diuretics are often indicated to control BP and avoid heart failure in people with chronic kidney disease, particularly when compliance is poor regarding sodium and fluid intake limits.

It has been said (an old Italian expression, we think) that "too much is sometimes like too little." Salt clearly fits this statement. Too little salt intake can paradoxically cause BP to rise because of a cascade of hormonal events. This can occur even if blood volume is contracted by excessive restriction of salt; of course, if blood volume is contracted too much, BP will decrease substantially, even to shock levels, but the hormonal cascade continues, even worsens. The kidneys respond to excessively decreased salt intake (whether a decrease in blood volume or serum sodium/chloride or all occur) by secreting a hormone called renin (not to be confused with an enzyme called rennin that causes milk to clot). Renin leads to production of a vasoconstrictor called angiotensin-II which increases BP through direct vasoconstriction of one's arteries and also causes the adrenal glands to secrete aldosterone, a hormone that causes the kidneys to reabsorb or conserve urinary sodium at the expense of potassium. Another hormone from the pituitary gland, called antidiuretic hormone or vasopressin, causes the kidneys to reabsorb water from the urine. The end point, here, is to recover blood volume or serum sodium/chloride levels or all of the foregoing. One definitely does not want to excite this "Renin-Angiotensin-Aldosterone Axis", particularly if one already has atherosclerosis. Aldosterone can cause serum potassium levels to decline markedly, due to an exchange of sodium for potassium in the kidneys, and this, along with high serum levels of angiotensin-II and aldosterone, may have a sclerosing effect on arteries, even small ones, over and above that due to atherosclerosis. Not having enough potassium in one's bloodstream is also not a good thing as this can lead to cardiac arrhythmias, even death from ventricular fibrillation. Conversely, if serum potassium is excessively high due to chronic kidney disease, the heart can be slowed to a standstill and cause death. So, it is best to keep both serum sodium and potassium levels within reasonable bounds, e.g., 135-145 mmol/l and 3.8-5.0 mmol/l, respectively.

Too much salt intake on a chronic basis, on the other hand, can also lead to an increase in BP because of blood and interstitial fluid volume expansion. If one has normal kidney function, the best pathway to health and the target levels of salt intake expressed above is to eat what is known as a "no added salt diet." That is, do not add table salt to any food that already has salt placed in it when being cooked. This certainly applies to any food eaten outside of one's home and, perhaps, in one's home, if the cook has a free hand with salt. Almost all restaurant foods and all processed foods will have excess salt in them. A thing to remember about salt is that "the more salt one eats, the more salt one has to eat in order to taste it." The threshold for the taste of salt moves up or down with the amount of salt eaten on a chronic basis. Finally, as indicated earlier, the chloride of salt imposes a significant acid burden; if for no other reason, salt should not be abused because of this. As indicated earlier, excessive salt intake may be a factor contributing to development of osteoporosis. Take the salt shaker off the dining table but leave the pepper shaker.

1.23 A rationale for targeted therapy

Risk of adverse therapeutic events weighed against benefits of therapy must always be taken into account, regardless of whether a physician is in the camp of "treat-to-target," "fire-and-forget" or "tailored treatment." Where potential benefit is concerned, again, it must be recognized that the production of oxidized LDL nanoparticles represents a "systems-biology weakness" due to excessive CHO intake, high arterial BP, and the high O_2 atmosphere of arterial blood. LDL nanoparticle numbers and size can be dealt with therapeutically, while the high O_2 atmosphere cannot, short of moving to a high altitude. And, in the important objective of controlling arterial BP, it can at best only be normalized without encountering side effects. In our opinion, even a "normal BP" remains a "significant BP" to some extent where atherosclerosis is concerned. We recommend proper diet as the initial form of therapy for most people and the use of a statin as adjunct therapy only if needed.

The Body Mass Index (BMI -- kg of body weight divided by height in m^2) is often used to rank people by size. People who are of normal weight (BMI 18-25 kg/m^2) will only need to change their macronutrient intake mix to meet recommendations for controlling VLDL and LDL production. People who are overweight (BMI > 25 kg/m^2), obese (BMI > 30 kg/m^2) or morbidly obese (BMI > 35 kg/m^2) will all likely have excessive *ectopic lipogenesis* of their striated muscle cells and liver cells and the potential for insulin resistance will be very high. This interferes significantly with both fatty acid and glucose oxidative metabolism throughout the body but certainly in liver and muscle cells. It is probably best, particularly for the overweight to morbidly obese, to initiate diet therapy first to provoke weight loss over a period say of 4-6 months before contemplating the need for statin therapy. Substantial weight loss will return muscle cell metabolism to a more normal state before initiating statin therapy which, as we speculate, may reduce the incidence of potential adverse effects of statins on one's musculature. Moreover, substantial weight loss, if needed, and movement of one's lipid factors in the proper direction may allow a patient to respond well to an inexpensive generic statin at a low or intermediate dose, e.g., fluvastatin (Lescol XL) or pravastatin (Pravachol), if needed, and avoid the major cost of a nongeneric statin. We have not observed anyone else linking diet and statin therapy in the way described here but we think it makes sense to do so. If, on the other hand, one does exhibit muscle problems on use of any of the cheaper generics, now including atorvastatin (Lipitor), he/she is likely to tolerate rosuvastatin (Crestor) quite well and, at the same time, gain an appreciably greater reduction in LDL though at much greater financial cost.

It is sometimes necessary to withhold statin dosing for a period of time and then rechallenge the patient with the same or another statin to make sure any muscle aches and pains are due to statin therapy. Major increases, i.e., greater than 10x's normal, in serum creatine phosphokinase (CPK) blood level indicate the presence of marked rhabdomyolysis (muscle destruction), as described below. Statin therapy must be withheld until the issue of rhabdomyolysis with resultant myoglobinemia totally clears and a decision will have to be made regarding a change in statin selection, if diet, alone, proves unsuccessful. However, if diet works well enough, don't worry about prescribing a statin. Diet control of LDL in patients who cannot tolerate statins is preferred, in our opinion, rather than current drug alternatives to statins. This would be particularly true also for people who experience cognitive impairment when taking a statin, a complication far less common and less appreciated than the myopathy issue. It would also be true for post-menopausal women who are ostensibly placed at greater risk of developing T2DM if treated with a statin.

The best approach, when administering a statin, is to dose incrementally over time to reach the target LDL level while watching for side effects when performing serial lipid and other studies (e.g., serum CPK levels if having muscle aches and pains). Other than obtaining pretreatment liver enzyme levels, recurrent liver enzyme determinations during statin therapy are no longer a requirement because statin related liver injury is so rare. Pretreatment enzyme levels are used to unwittingly avoid treating someone with a statin who has acute liver failure or decompensated cirrhosis. Where older patients are concerned, it may be a good idea to obtain a pretreatment serum thyroid stimulating hormone (TSH) level, as hypothyroidism can worsen the issue of muscle pain when taking a statin. Hypothroidism, itself, can cause muscle pain. In general, the older statins such as fluvastatin (Lescol XL), cerivastatin (Baycol – off the market because of rhabdomyolysis problems), pravastatin (Pravachol), and simvastatin (Zocor) do not possess the efficacy of the two somewhat newer statins such as atorvastatin (Lipitor) and rosuvastatin (Crestor, comes off patent in 2016). Moreover, particularly when compared to rosuvastatin (Crestor), when raised to maximum dose, the older statins increase their tendency to adversely affect one's musculature while only modestly improving LDL control. In fact, simvastatin (Zocor), according to recent 2011 FDA instructions, can no longer be used at its maximum daily dose of 80 mg to treat new patients because it so commonly causes muscle problems, particularly rhabdomyolysis, at this dosage. There is one exception among the generic statins, fluvastatin (Lescol XL); it can be used at maximum dose without much greater risk for muscle problems but unfortunately not at very much greater efficacy in reducing LDL concentration. We have purposefully avoided mention of drugs such as fibrates, niacin and bile salt sequesters that can be used either in conjunction with or in lieu of statins. As a class, fibrates, particularly phenofibrate, don't offer much improvement in lipid levels but they do increase the risk of muscle problems, particularly within the diabetic population and they can cause (reversible?) reduction in kidney function. The fibrates, including phenofibrate, can worsen kidney function particularly in people who already have chronic kidney disease and in the elderly. Niacin is not tolerated well by most patients for a variety of reasons, including the niacin induced "flush" and liver problems caused by the slow release varieties of niacin that avoid the "flush." Bile salt sequesters lack efficacy probably because, in most people, the liver enhances its production of cholesterol in response to cholesterol lost via the GI tract. Sequesters are also not generally well tolerated by patients.

Muscle issues can be grouped into three categories of increasing severity: myalgia (muscle pain), myositis (indicates inflammation but there is no sign of this on muscle biopsy) and rhabdomyolysis (muscle destruction, serum CPK > 10x's normal), a serious problem as this can lead to kidney failure and other health issues. Muscle problems, collectively speaking, are probably much more common in the real world of patient therapy, as typified by the following incidences of: 5.1% (fluvastatin); 10.9% (pravastatin); 14.9% (atorvastatin); and, 18.2% (simvastatin). The randomized controlled trials used to test statin efficacy screen patients extensively for muscle disorders and affected patients are not utilized in such studies if positive for chronic muscle aches and pains.[41]

Thus, irrespective of one's personal or family related risk factors for atherosclerosis, we recommend the following target levels after a 12-14 hr overnight fast, whether or not one is drug naïve for a statin:

- Total Cholesterol level of $\leq$ 150 mg/dl
- Triglyceride level of $\leq$ 70 mg/dl
- HDL cholesterol level of $\geq$ 70 mg/dl
- VLDL cholesterol level of $\leq$ 15 mg/dl
- LDL cholesterol level $\geq$ 25 but $\leq$ 50 mg/dl

The target values listed above are based on using current laboratory technology which, unfortunately, does not typically include particle number and size distribution analysis of LDL. Small, oxidized LDL is atherogenic while large LDL is less so, if at all. One must remember that the LDL in mg/dl usually seen on a lipid report is commonly a calculated, i.e., an estimated, value expressed by the Friedewald Equation [LDL, mg/dl = Tot. Chol. – (HDL + 0.2TRIG)]. Some insight into LDL size can be gained from calculating the TRIG/HDL ratio, particularly in Caucasians but not so reliably in African-Americans. A ratio of < 2.0 signals that the amount of small dense LDL is minimal, while a ratio > 2.0 suggests an increase in small, dense atherogenic LDL. The same relationship of the ratio also can be used to predict the presence or absence of insulin resistance.

In the future, the LDL CHOL target level may move downward to the > 25 but < 50 mg/dl range we propose for everyone in need of treatment which would then likely reduce concern over number and size of the LDL particles. Notably, as mentioned earlier, people with the heterozygous genetic disorder known as hypobetalipoproteinemia have been observed to have total CHOL levels of around 80 mg/dl and LDL CHOL levels of around 30 mg/dl without any obvious ill effects, particularly in their ability to absorb fat soluble vitamins. The < 50 mg/dl LDL target level recommended today by the National Cholesterol Education Program for people with multiple risk factors is clearly safe and achievable for people without "risk factor justification." In our opinion, the decision to treat should be based on "laboratory justification" first and other factors second because atherosclerosis is an insidious disease and often difficult to diagnose before an apocalyptic event occurs years later after the initial observation. We recommend safe dietary measures first and statin therapy second, if needed. A lower LDL level can probably be achieved by not eating fruits and berries or consuming alcohol. However, consumption of fruits and berries can be justified, healthwise, for a number of reasons; moreover, their exclusion is not necessary to reach the target levels listed above. Their exclusion from one's diet could prove quite unhealthful in the long run for a variety of reasons. Moderating alcohol intake is a realistic and important goal for most people who imbibe, if the subject of drinking alcohol is approached correctly in a multi-factorial way.

Unfortunately, chylomicron levels are never present on the standard lipid report. Hence, we do not have direct quantitative insight into the impact of the long-chain fatty acids we eat, these being the likely culprits in generalized insulin resistance. Chylomicrons do not directly affect LDL levels. However, their fatty acids can recirculate to the liver from nonliver tissues and be included by this indirect route in VLDL produced through DNL in the liver. So, in the broadest sense, VLDL derived from the liver's pool of fatty acids and separately plasma TRIG's could be considered surrogate markers for how well chylomicrons are cleared from one's bloodstream. The value of the VLDL and TRIG as surrogates for chylomicron levels is obviously related to how much fructose, glucose and alcohol one consumes. The target value for VLDL of ≤ 15 mg/dl and plasma TRIG of ≤ 70 mg/dl proposed above, however, indirectly tells one that his/her clearance of chylomicrons is very likely quite adequate. The implication, here, is that the intake of long-chain fatty acids is unlikely to be excessive relative to need. The large size of chylomicrons is directly related to the amount of TRIG's of long-chain fatty acids one consumes at each meal. If difficulty is incurred in reducing TRIG levels, then supplemental Omega-3 oils are often quite helpful in doing so and they also help elevate one's HDL level somewhat, as well. Because of their high degree of unsaturation, they tend to make LDL of a larger size that is probably not atherogenic.

We believe physicians must learn to start treatment at an early enough patient age, say in the 20-30 year age range, as opposed to suddenly embarking on treating middle aged people to reverse their lifetimes of over indulgence. If there is reticence about treating only numbers, then an external carotid US and a coronary EBCT can be considered in making the determination of whether to initiate treatment or not. There is nothing wrong with waiting to treat but this includes only the use of statins, not diet. It is interesting that new NIH guidelines call for screening dyslipidemia in children initially between ages 9-11 years and in follow up between ages 17-21 years. It is estimated that up to 60% of children with dyslipidemia may be missed if screening is based only on a family history of dyslipidemia or premature cardiovascular disease. The issue always is whether or not to treat young people with a statin because ostensibly one is looking at a lifetime of therapy. Really long term untoward effects of statins, if any, are unknown, level of compliance over decades would be hard to assess, and it is unknown whether treating children will prevent future cardiovascular disease. It is always difficult to treat someone who might be asymptomatic but the physician has to be able to look decades into the younger patient's future to determine the importance of therapy. This includes treating LDL levels above the target value, with diet first and a statin second or both concomitantly, if age, lipid values, personal history, diet, alcohol consumption, smoking, physical exam, family history, and other findings merit it. Obviously, the diet we recommend, sans statin therapy, would be of great help in reversing dyslipidemia and would not be harmful by any account, if kidney function is reasonable.

If the above approach is followed, we may well save a lot more people from the ravages of aggressive atherosclerosis in middle age, that 40-70 middle-age group referred to earlier. This is particularly important when one considers the rising tide in the U.S. of overweight and obese children and adolescents that is steadily but surely fostering huge numbers of people without "clinically" apparent atherosclerosis as they move into early adulthood. As for the elderly (defined here as people > 75 years of age), we see no reason not to implement diet therapy if the LDL is > 50 or if there is clinical evidence of atherosclerotic disease, particularly if it involves either the heart or the brain or both. If significant atherosclerosis exists, adding an inexpensive generic statin, if needed, at low dose, is clearly a reasonable option, assuming the individual is otherwise alert, comprehending, mobile, performs daily activities without difficulty and is not having difficulty remembering when and what to take, if polypharmacy already exists.

It appears that at LDL levels of < 70 mg/dl[2] and for sure at levels of < 50 mg/dl[42], atherosclerosis can be subdued, even reversed. However, if the atherosclerotic lesions are already advanced in size, heavily calcified and the large and medium size arteries are dilated before therapy is initiated, as is often the case in the middle-age group, many of the vascular changes that have already occurred remain, along with the dense calcium deposition and perhaps a latent risk for an adverse cardiovascular event. What becomes absent in the treatment of the older (and the younger) age group with proper diet and statin, if the latter is needed, is silent vascular inflammation. This is probably the most important achievement as it leads to reduction or avoidance of growth of atheromata, both in size and in numbers. A reduction in inflammation allows the BMDACs, spoken to earlier, to repair/remodel damaged endothelium more effectively in order to maintain endothelial integrity and stabilization. In the range of 25-50 mg/dl for LDL, the innate immune system can clearly manage the burden of oxidized LDL particles in the subendothelial spaces. The approach outlined here offers primary prevention of atherosclerosis and it is unlikely to impact fat soluble vitamin absorption or pose any other negative metabolic threat, short or long term.

We are aware of how relative risk and risk reduction are considered in the real world. There is a government sponsored National Cholesterol Education Program link on the internet to a "10-year heart attack risk calculator". Risk numbers are often missrepresented by drug companies. For example, if one's risk is estimated to be 1% in 10 years, that means one person in 100 in a time frame of 10 years will have a heart attack. Such risk calculations are based on total CHOL, HDL, age, gender, smoking status, BP status and medications. Thus, if one's risk is 1%, this means that in 300 people, three people would be at risk of having a heart attack even if taking a statin. If one of the three doesn't have a heart attack, this is interpreted to mean that the statin has lowered the risk of having a heart attack by about a third. The other two taking a statin did have a heart attack in spite of taking the drug. The other 297 people remaining would not have had a heart attack even though they were not taking the drug. The point is that, when represented as a 33% reduction in heart attack relative risk, it is a marketing ploy. The implication is that one is at 100% risk before taking a drug when 297 not on a statin did not experience a heart attack in 10 years and they would not have benefited from statin therapy in this regard. That would provide a huge pool of people to treat with a statin to save one person from having a heart attack where this complication is concerned.

But, the issues are not just heart attacks; the problem is cardiovascular disease which means all larger arteries are at risk of atherosclerosis, not just the coronaries. The risk issues include, in addition to heart attacks, strokes, ruptured aneurysms and peripheral vascular disease. This is particularly true if one is overweight or obese which strongly implies that one imbibes excessive amounts of fructose, glucose and perhaps alcohol relative to need. And, again, cardiovascular disease is a silent process until the apocalypse occurs and its presence can be very difficult to establish pre-emptively unless invasive studies are done, such as an intravascular US study or a noninvasive EBCT of the coronaries or other vessels. This is why dietary intervention, at a minimum, is so important, not just intervention with a medication.

One must also appreciate that 10 years is not a very long time when considering progression of atherosclerosis unless one is older. There is a major difference in the clinical extent of this problem when examining people in the 20-30 decade compared to those in the 60-70 decade. The ground work for atherosclerosis in the latter decade rests on the eating habits of the prior 60 to 70 years but only the prior 20 to 30 years in the former decade. If one waits for the apocalypse to occur to signify the presence of atherosclerosis, then the issue of atherosclerosis can become much more difficult to deal with medically in older people and it will more likely be a medically-related cause of death. In a sense, the 1% is as misleading as the 33%. Again, diet moves to the forefront in prevention.

Are there new drugs in the pipeline to treat LDL cholesterol? There always are and probably always will be. One of the more admirable new approaches features a human monoclonal antibody, REGN727, to PCSK9, a serine protease enzyme that regulates LDL receptor expression throughout the body. High circulating levels of PCSK9 cause depletion of LDL receptors and this directly interferes with clearing LDL nanoparticles from the bloodstream. Statins, on the other hand, increase the liver's expression of LDL nanoparticle receptors but unfortunately they also increase the release of the PCSK9 protease enzyme into the systemic circulation that causes a total body decrease in LDL receptors. This counter regulatory action of statins on PCSK9 is one of the main factors that blunt the effectiveness of statins. The antibody to PCSK9, REGN727, binds and blocks circulating PCSK9 and, therefore, has a much greater LDL lowering action than statins. Intravenous injection of the antibody appears to be more effective than subcutaneous injection. The drug is now in phase 2 trials and so far has exhibited minimal toxic side effects. The authors of the study suggest that REGN727 would be most effective if used in conjunction with diet.[43] We couldn't agree more where diet is concerned but it is premature to consider the drug to be more than a novelty at this time because it will have to go through both phase 3 and long term toxicity testing once dosed in "real world" patients. It is interesting that people who lack PCSK9 production due to a monogenic defect have LDL nanoparticle levels of about 15 mg/dl without any adverse effects and little or no atherosclerosis. This dovetails with our recommendations of 25-50 mg/dl blood levels for LDL.

In our opinion, cost will likely be a major limiting factor in the use of a human monoclonal antibody on a chronic basis, particularly if it has to be given intravenously because this means a visit to the doctor's office at some frequency in addition to whatever the likely major direct cost of this drug will be to the consumer. Moreover, this medication does not alter eating habits or achieve weight loss if needed. At this juncture, we believe that our dietary recommendations, alone or with a statin, if needed, would prove most efficacious for the vast majority of people with a LDL nanoparticle problem at an extremely low cost.

Finally, a recent article involving the role of monocytes in atherosclerosis relates that chemokines have been identified which control the entry and exit of monocytes into the subendothelial space. Macrophages express netrin-1, and one of its receptors, Unc5b, which blocks the egress of macrophages from inflamed vessel walls in the presence of hypercholesterolemia. Such egress is otherwise prompted by the chemokine, CCL2. Lowering CHOL enhances egress of the macrophages. Both netrin-1 and Unc5b are expressed in macrophages within human arterial plaques. Their expression is enhanced by CHOL loading in both human and mouse macrophages. The authors suggest that this finding (increased expression of netrin-1 and Unc5b) indicates a potential mechanism for increasing the egress of macrophages if the netrin-1 effect can be blocked.[44] We suggest that this might not be advisable, if oxidized LDL nanoparticles are present at high levels. It simply baits the question: What would happen to all of the oxidized LDL? Our feeling continues that the LDL issue is a mass balance problem that is resolved best through dietary means. Besides, it appears that lowering cholesterol through diet helps clear the macrophages from the sub-endothelial space.

We repeat. It is fructose, glucose and alcohol that turn on DNL and the production of VLDL which leads to the production of the so called LDL CHOL. The CHOL is just a passenger on the LDL nanoparticles as are PL and TRIG's. CHOL does not control DNL. The CHO's we discuss in this text are also the factors that cause oxidation of LDL nanoparticles.

References

1. Pollan, Michael. *The New York Times Magazine.* "Mysteries Solved, Riddles Explained, and Readers' Questions Answered." p. 34 (10/2/2011).

2. Esselstyn, Caldwell B., Jr., M.D. *Prevent and Reverse Heart Disease.* Penguin Group: Avery, 2007.

3. *The Week. The Best of the U.S. and International Media.* "The Bottom Line." P. 39 (Nov. 11, 2011).

4. Hansson, Goran K., M.D., Ph.D. "Mechanisms of Disease – Inflammation, Atherosclerosis, and Coronary Artery Disease." *NEJM* (April 21, 2005) 352; 16: 1685-1695.

5. Lloyd-Jones D, Adams RJ, Brown TM, et al. "Heart Disease and Stroke Statistics – 2010 update: a report from the American Heart Association." *Circulation* 2010; 121(7):e46-e215.

6. Dreier, Frederick (2011, August 7) "Death During Swim Renews Questions About Events Safety." *The New York Times on the Web.* Retrieved December 10, 2011, from http:/www.nytimes.com/2011/08/08. "sports/man-dies-during-new-york-city-triathlon." html

7. Grant, Michael. *The Courier Journal.* Sports, p. C1, Winner of 1st triathlon here scores an impressive victory; Louisville, KY: Monday, August 29, 2011.

8. Allen, Jane E. (2011, November 21) Adrenaline-Fueled Sprint Makes Some Marathons Deadly. Retrieved December 10, 2011. From http://abcnews.go.com/HealthHeart Disease/marathondeaths/story?id=15000378/2011/2011/11/21

9. Erardi, John. *The Cincinnati Enquirer.* "Back from the 'dead',Dave will run today." p. A1. Thursday, November 24, 2011.

10. Kim, J.H, et al. "Cardiac Arrest during Long-Distance Running Races." *NEJM* (January 12, 2012) 366; 2: 130-140.

11. Albano, Alfred J., Thompson, Paul D., and Kapur, Navin K. "Acute Coronary Thrombosis in Boston Marathon Runners." NEJM (January 12, 2012) (correspondence); 366; 2:184-185.

12. Browning, Jeffrey D. and Holton, Jay D. "Molecular mediators of hepatic steatosis and liver injury." *J. Clin. Invest.* (July 15, 2004); 114; 2:147-152.

13. Lustig, Robert H. Fructose: "Metabolic, Hedonic, and Societal Parallels with Ethanol." *Journal of the American Dietetic Association.* (2010) 110; 1307-1321.

14. Dekker, M.J., Qiaozhu, Su, Baker, C., Rutledge, A. C., and Adeli, K. "Fructose: a highly lipogenic nutrient implicated in insulin resistance, hepatic steatosis, and the metabolic syndrome." *Am J Physiol Endocrinol Metab.* 299: E685-E694,2010. First published September 7, 2010; doi:101152/ ajpendo.00283.2010.

15. Kyriazis, G. A., Soundarapandian, M.M., and Tyrberg, B.: "Sweet Taste Receptor Signaling in Beta Cells Mediates Fructose-induced Potentiation of Glucose Stimulated

Insulin Secretion." *Science News*, Vol. 177, March 27, 2010, p. 22. Published online Feb. 6, 2012. doi:10.1073/pnas.1115183109.

16. Johner, S.A., Libuda, I., Shi, I, Retzlaff, A., Joslowsli, G., and Remer, T.: "Urinary fructose: a potential biomarker for dietary fructose intake in children." *European Journal of Clinical Nutrition.* (2010) 64; 1365-1370. Doi:10.1038/ejcn. 2010.160.

17. Rutledge, A. C. and Adeli, K.: "Fructose and the metabolic syndrome: pathophysiology and molecular mechanisms." *Nutrition Reviews.* (June 2007) 65;6: S13-S23.

18. Tonkonogi, M. and Salin, K. "Physical exercise and mitochondrial function in human skeletal muscle." *Exerc Sport Sci Rev.* (2002) 30: 129-137.

19. Palmieri, F. "The mitochondrial transporter family (SLC25): Physiological and pathological implications." *Pflugers Arch.* (2004) 447: 689-709.

20. http://themedicalbiochemistrypage.org/glycolysis.html. p.10.

21. Parks, Elizabeth J., Skokan, L.E., Timlin, M.T., and Dingfelder, C.S. "Dietary sugars stimulate fatty acid synthesis in adults." *J. Nutri.* (2008) 138:1039-1046.

22. Ginsberg, H.N. and Goldberg, I. J. "Disorders of Lipoprotein Metabolism." Chapt. 344; 2245-2257. *Harrison's Principles of Internal Medicine*, 15th Ed. McGraw Hill, 2001.

23. Siler, S. Q., Neese, R.A., and Hellerstein, M.K. "De novo lipogenesis, lipid kinetics and whole-body lipid balances in humans after acute alcohol consumption." *Am. J. Clin. Nutr.* (1999) 70: 928-936.

24. Hellerstein, M.K., Christiansen, M., Kaempfer, S., Kletke, C., Wu, K., Reid, J.S., Mulligan, K., Hellerstein, N.S., and Shackleton, C. H., "Measurement of de novo hepatic lipogenesis in humans using stable isotopes." *J. Clin. Invest.* (1991) 87:1841-1852.

25. Schwarz, J.M., Linfoot, P., Dare, D., amd Aghajanian, K. "Hepatic de novo lipogenesis in normoinsulinemic and hyperinsulinemic subjects consuming high fat, low carbohydrate and low fat, high carbohydrate isoenergetic diets." *Am. J. Clin. Nutr.* (2003) 77: 43-50.

26. Donnelly, K. L., Smith, C.I., Schwarzenberg, S. J., Jessurun, J., Boldt, M.D., and Parks, E.J. "Sources of fatty acids stored in the liver and secreted via lipoproteins in patients with nonalcoholic fatty liver disease." *J. Clin. Invest.* (2005) 115: 1343-1351.

27. Hudgins, L.C., Hellerstein, M.K., Seidman, C.E., Neese, R.A., Tremaroli, J.D, and Hirsch, J. "Relationship between carbohydrate-induced hypertriglyceri-demia and fatty acid synthesis in lean and obese subjects." *J. Lipid Res.* (2000) 41: 595-604.

28. Schwarz, J.M., Noworolski, S.M., Lee, G.A., Wen, M., Dyachenko, A., Prior, J., Weinberg, M., Herraiz, L., Rao, M., and Mulligan, K. "Effects of short-term feeding with high- vs low-fructose isoenergetic diets on hepatic de novo lipogenesis, liver fat content and glucose regulation." *Diabetes.* (2009) 1476P. abstr.

29. Havel, Peter J. "Dietary fructose: Implications for dysregulation of energy homeostasis and lipid/carbohydrate metabolism." *Nutrition Reviews* (2005) 63; 5: 133-157.

30a. Olofsson, S., Bostrom , P., Lagerstedt, J., Andersson, L., Adiels, M., Perman, J., Rutberg, M. Lu, L., and Boren, J. Chapt. 1, pp 1-26. "The lipid droplet: A dynamic organelle, not only involved in the storage and turnover of lipids." *Cellular Lipid Metabolism*, Ehnholm, C., Editor (Springer, 2009).

30b. Olkkonen, Vesa M. Chapt 2, pp 27-71. "Oxysterols and Oxysterol-Binding Proteins in Cellular Lipid Metabolism." *Cellular Lipid Metabolism*, Ehnholm. C., Editor (Srpinger, 2009).

31. www.health.harvard.edu, Sept 2011. Harvard Heart Letter, p. 5.

32. Jung, S. L., Mietus-Snyder, M., Valente, A., Schwarz, J., and Lustig, R. H. "The role of fructose in the pathogenesis of NAFLD and the metabolic syndrome." *Nature Reviews/Gastroenterology & Hepatology.* (May 2010) 7: 251-264.

33. McGavock, Jonathan M., Victor, Ronald G., Unger, Roger H., and Szczepaniak, Lidia, S.: "Adiposity of the Heart, Revisited." *Ann. Int. Med.* (2006) 144: 517-524.

34. Ritman, Erik, : and Lerman, Amir. "The dynamic vaso vasorum." *Cardiovasc. Res.* (September 1, 2007) 75;4: 649-658.

35. Semenza, G. L. "Mechanisms of disease: Oxygen sensing, homeostatis and disease." *NEJM* (August 11, 2011) 365;6: 537-547.

36. Feng Xia Ma, Bin Zhou, Zhong Chen, Qian Ren, Shi Hong Lu, Tatsuya Sawamura, and Zhong Chao Han. "Oxidized low density lipoprotein impairs endothelial progenitor cells by regulation of endothelial nitric oxide synthase." *J. of Lipid Research* (March 7, 2006) 47: 1227-1237.

37. Singh, Vibhuti N. "Low LDL Cholestesterol (Hypobetalipoproteinemia)." http://emedicine.medscape.com/article/121975-overview. Updated Aug.4, 2009.

38. Hampton, Beverly G. and Bryant, Ruth A. "Ostomies and content diversions." *Nursing management.* Mosby Year Book (1992) P. 291.

39. High Density Lipoprotein. http://en.wikipedia.org/wiki/high density lipo-protein.

40. Cordain, Loren. *The Paleo Diet* (Wiley, 2011). pp. 11 (diet) and 128-129 (nuts).

41. Fernandez, Genaro, Spatz, Erica S., Jablecki, Charles, and Phillips, Paul S. "Statin myopathy: A common dilemma not reflected in clinical trials." *Cleveland Clinic J. of Med.* (June 2011) 78;6: 393-403.

42. O'Keefe, jr., James H., Cordain, Loren, Harris, William H., Moe, Richard M., and Vogel, Robert. "Optimal Low-Density Lipoprotein is 50 to 70 mg/dl." *J. of the American College of Cardiology.* (June 2, 2004) 43;11: 2142-2146.

43. Stein, Evan A., et al. "Effect of a Monoclonal Antibody to PCSK9 on LDL Cholesterol." *NEJM* (March 22, 2012). 366; 12: 1108.

44. Gerszten, Robert E. and Tager, Andrew M. "The Monocyte in Atherosclerosis — Should I Stay or Go Now?" *NEJM* (May 3, 2012) 366; 18: 1734.

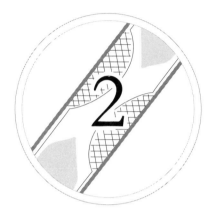

Section Two
A Psychological Scientific Approach to Diet

Introduction

In Section 1 of this book we provided the scientific rationale and a method for mitigating the eventually fatal condition, atherosclerosis. In the process, we also showed how natural processes of the human body can avoid what we call the "way point" or non-communicable diseases (NCD's) of atherosclerosis: overweight, obesity, kidney disease, diabetes, and hypertension.

What we provided was based on the integration of many years of accumulated scientific evidence plus the insights that we have had both in professional practice and in reviewing the scientific evidence. The sum of our position is that atherosclerosis can be mitigated and that diseases related to it can be prevented through proper diet and lifestyle.

We strongly believe that this is a positive finding. We have been very pleased with our finding that the wisdom of the ages has been confirmed repeatedly over time. Hippocrates viewed food and medicine as opposite sides of the same coin. In its many thousands of years of evolution the human body has become exquisitely adapted to its natural environment. Our difficulties today do not seem to be due to nature but instead are due to the way that man has modified natural substances. We cited the example of fructose. In its natural form and quantity to be found in fruits, fructose is essentially harmless and also beneficial due to the antioxidants and other micronutrients that are always found with it in the natural setting such as a blueberry. When fructose is modified and available in a very highly concentrated form, fructose is not only toxic but it is the leading cause of atherosclerosis and the other NCD's listed in Section 1. Fructose is at the root of the most serious epidemics that western man, and increasingly man generally, face today.

In no case do we imply that modern medicines are not useful and needed. However, we endorse the wisdom of the late Herman C.B. Denber[45] that there are no safe medicines. There are only safe doctors. Also we have come to reject some of the implications of a company's slogan of some years ago: better things for better living, through chemistry. We should not be turning first to chemistry. Our first look should be at what the human body is adapted to at this stage of its evolution. We should give it that. After we have done so, we may begin a fruitful exploration of what science can do for the human body that the human body cannot do adequately for itself. Always we must be guided by that most ancient of medical instructions: first, do no harm.

For many readers Section 1 will be all they need in order to benefit from the science that is behind eat right for your height (ERFYH). They will embrace ERFYH principles and they will receive the rewards for doing so. They will recognize the rationale and they will figure out a way to get around any obstacles to reaching their goal. We applaud those who can do that. If need be, any such reader may return to Section 1 and take from it what he or she needs in order to make reaching personal goals in his or her own way go better.

A supplemental perspective

There are some readers who will want or need more. We are happy to provide that in Section 2 of this book. We have chosen one well researched approach to making ERFYH work. We trust that no reader will need more than we provide but just in case we have also provided a bibliography (Appendix A) that will guide personal research into the area.

In a very real sense Section 2 itself provides a supplemental perspective. For those who want or need more than what Section 1 provides it is here to be used. It may even be that using the materials to be found in Section 2 will be helpful to anyone because of the powerful method that we are recommending. We want to make very clear that Section 1 provides everything that one may need from the scientific point of view. Knowing and applying what is in Section 1 will lead to success in dealing with overweight or obesity and mitigating atherosclerosis. If there is a trick to Section 1 as many seem to wish for, it is in the application of Section 1 to one's own personal nature and conditions. What we choose to do has to fit us.

In Section 1, we reviewed a wide variety of literature from medical and other sources. This knowledge was scattered around and was piecemeal in its approach. This reflects the nature of scientific inquiry and its rules for discovery in part. We have had to sift through this and find a way to separate wheat from chaff. What we found is what is in this book. We recommend that the reader use what we discovered as a foundation. We recommend even more strongly that our view summarized as ERFYH or "Eat Right For Your Height" be integrated into the reader's more or less automatic way of looking at his world or what can be called his assumptive world according to psychiatrist Jerome Frank.[46] ERFYH is the best we have and it represents our many years of study. We see no reason for the reader to re-invent the wheel. If what we are offering is taken into one's assumptive world there will be a lot of room for other important insights to prevent becoming at cross purposes. We suggest that readers build on what we have done.

What we mean by an assumptive world again is the integrated set of beliefs that a person develops as he or she deals with what the psychologist William James[47] termed the blooming, buzzing confusion into which we are born. This aspect of a human being's cognition evolves over time. It is not easy to alter it but it can be altered. We construct it and we can change it.

If one is to use ERFYH successfully it is essential to deal with whatever assumptive world that one brings to the situation that needs altering. By becoming one's own personal scientist, it is possible to alter strongly held beliefs or attitudes that sorely need to be addressed. If one views the overweight or obese as losers or hopelessly weak of will but also knows that objectively he or she is overweight or obese that belief will prevent initial success at ERFYH. The essence of the corrective procedure is to collect evidence that will settle the question of whether one actually is a loser who cannot lose life threatening fat. More is required than simply telling the individual what one thinks such as "you may be fat right now but you are not a loser." As clinicians we have had to admit the painful truth that our saying such things does not help. Something more is needed and that something is Cognitive Behavioral Therapy.

The concept of the assumptive world includes the idea that belief drives behavior much as the philosopher and longshoreman Eric Hoffer taught us in his seminal book The True Believer.[48] We have found that what Hoffer, Frank,

James, and others have said is quite true. That clearly means that if belief drives behavior a change of belief must precede behavior change. It is but a small jump to conclude further that the individual's assumptive world is largely expressed in that individual's attitude.

Much of Section 2 is about a very well proven method of altering negative thoughts or cognitions and developing behaviors that are unquestionably indicative of success. We make no claim that what we recommend is unique to us. We can claim that ERFYH includes techniques that we have observed being successful for many years. We are certain that we are recommending what is today the very best way of implementing ERFYH.

What we have written in Section 2 is anchored in so many contributions by so many scholars and practitioners that it is impossible for us to acknowledge them all. We will instead pay our respects here to those courageous pioneers, the hunter-gatherers, who preceded us many millennia ago some of whom are still around today. They took the chance of sampling foods of all kinds from nature's bounty and determined whether they were toxic or safe. Who could know in advance that an apple or a mushroom could be safe? Someone had to try the substances and pass on their experience to others. Following this line of thinking, we can ask who that special person or group of persons was that figured out what fish were, what made them bite, and when to leave them alone. We owe a debt to those who came before us. We can repay that debt by accepting ERFYH and making it work for us.

There is always a core lesson that a study gives us. The one from this book is that we are capable of being healthy and long lived. Each of us has to make the choices that will make that capacity a reality.

2.2   *The think system for eat right for your height* (ERFYH)

Je pense donc je suis, (I think therefore I am)—Rene' Descartes, 1637. When most of us were exposed to the philosophy of Rene Descartes in any sort of formal way we most probably heard the Latin version of what he wrote: cogito, ergo sum.[49] rather than his earlier French version of the idea. One way or the other this idea is the basis for much of Western thought. It is equally the basis of one of the pillars of Cognitive Behavioral Therapy (CBT) which in turn is the psychological device that we use in this program. We take a slight liberty with what Descartes[50] said in that we emphasize human reasoning: I reason, therefore I am. This approach utilizes well accepted philosophy but it is just as well grounded in the work of O.H. Mowrer who was a giant in understanding cognitive processes in learning theory.[51] Whether we come from a background in philosophy or science, we come to the same place.

Our approach is slightly different in another way. Many years ago we were faced with explaining the integration of rigorous Behavior Therapy and the relatively new Cognitive Therapy to students from various disciplines. Our research group used the term Cognitive Behavior Therapy to emphasize this integration. In our teaching we also found it fruitful to use a term that we borrowed from the popular Broadway Musical *The Music Man* and apply it to the treatment of depression. The term that we used following Professor Harold Hill of that musical was "The Think System."

Recall that con man Hill persuaded town's people whom he was defrauding that their children needed no instruments at first in order to learn to play in the River City Boy's Band. He said that the boys just needed to think the playing and it would happen when it needed to happen. The first thing to do was to give the professor the money for the instruments which he had no intention of spending on musical instruments. Later and miraculously when Professor Hill's scalp was on the line he directed the band and the parents heard the boys playing everything just right with their finally received instruments. What the parents thought was so came to be. Such is the power not of miracles but of the human brain. What we human beings desperately want to hear we hear and we are certain that we heard it. Professor Harold Hill's approach has to be modified toward emphasis on the truth as we perfect our own version of ERFYH but it is what we think that will make it so.

Actually the citizens of River City were making the cognitive error that is known as faulty reasoning. This speaks loudly to the consequences of not being one's own personal scientist and sticking to the facts when it comes to food ingestion. What we eat is what it is no matter what we want it to be and the consequences can be much worse than being defrauded by a musical instrument con man. Faulty reasoning is the pathway to atherosclerosis and death.

Rational thought is extremely valuable in ERFYH. Rational thought is possible for the human being because of a comparatively tiny amount of the human brain. Yet it is this small amount of our brain that makes us human and along with the oppositional thumb has given us most of what we needed for dominance over every other species on earth. Our oppositional thumb has been the key to developing tools and adding to what our muscles allow us to do. Being capable of abstract thinking adds to what our brains are able to do. In remarkable ways we are able to go beyond the information that our environment gives us at any time and we are able to reason about what that information may mean. It has been demonstrated convincingly that other species apparently have some capacity for abstract reasoning but what the human being has is formidable by comparison.

Members of other species mostly are bound by reflex. When the environment presents them with information of a certain sort they react automatically and generally in their interest. They are dominated by a brain that is similar to the part of the human brain that causes us to blink involuntarily when a puff of air hits our eye. For millions of years this reflex dominated brain has allowed species to survive. In their own environment this reflex dominated brain does not turn against an individual's interests. They survive and they thrive.

It is not possible to overemphasize the value of having the additional ability to reason and go beyond the information given. Without doubt science is the most highly developed form of our reasoning capacity although we have others such as legal and theological reasoning that have helped us adapt. The formidable accomplishments of science are very clear. We will cite just two of them but we encourage you to take a few minutes to think about other accomplishments in your own lifetime. Can we even imagine that a reflex dominated brain could have reasoned from observation of the behavior of a mold (fungus) to the understanding of an antibiotic substance found in nature and then to ridding mankind of a scourge of infectious diseases? We speak of penicillin of course.

Is it remotely possible to imagine that a reflex dominated brain could have discovered the capacity to warp an airplane wing and have that capacity result in the intercontinental travel and shrinking globe we have today? Increasing the number of environments that a given group of human beings can live in as global travel has done is no small thing! Most species by contrast are limited to existence in a tiny fragment of earth. The glow worms of New Zealand caves flourish in those particular caves but would perish quickly if they were anywhere else. The examples of this phenomenon are endless.

When one takes on the task of ERFYH, one faces the probability of a very negative consequence of what Descartes said. "I reason therefore I am" can become "I reason in a faulty way and I have become something that is very dangerous for me." The original faulty reasoning often leads to very destructive thoughts, behaviors, and conditions. Individuals and even large groups can be destroyed by such faulty reasoning related to food intake. If we look around us we will see rampant malignant obesity that is resulting in equally rampant diabetes, atherosclerotic heart disease, and hip and other joint problems that were almost unknown until recent decades. Our biology has not changed much during these decades. The amount of our reasoning about food intake that is faulty has become equally epidemic. What has changed for the human being in a few decades has not changed for other species in a million years of natural evolution.

You may ask: How this can be? Just how can our rationality destroy us? It is quite simple. If we look at species that have reflex dominated brains we find that they ingest certain foods from all of the possible foods in their environment and these are the foods that have proved best for them over time. It has become automatic. When confronted by a nearby fly, a frog gets it with a flip of his tongue. The macronutrients that the frog needs are neatly packaged in that food. We can observe the frog for months on end in its natural environment and we will never see that frog take in a macronutrient that is not appropriate for him.

Now shift to the behavior of the human being. His capacity for reasoning also includes the capacity for faulty reasoning. Section 1 made clear that we are just as needy as the frog is for just the right macronutrients. We are as capable of learning this as frogs are and science has given us that knowledge. We have so much mobility and adaptability that we can live almost anywhere. There is no need for us to be limited to a specific environment or method that provides those macronutrients. Because we can move around we can use that capacity to get to where the proper food for us is located. Science has allowed us to know precisely what we need and our task is only to ferret out what we need in any environment. If it is not in the environment where we are, we can carry it with us even if we go into space. We know that even without science the history of mankind has included the development of food habits or diets that give us just what we need. Without science it is true that every food habit that man has developed in every culture except one has provided an excellent balance of the macronutrients (PROT, FAT, CHO) and the micronutrients that are needed for health. The only requirement is that the nutrients be those that can be found in nature.

It is faulty reasoning that leads us to ingest substances that are not right for us and it is faulty reasoning that allows us to poison ourselves or gorge ourselves while telling ourselves that we are not doing just that. Unlike a frog we have the capacity literally to eat ourselves to death. While doing so we may not be at all aware that we are behaving in this suicidal way. The reasons for what we do to ourselves are a bit complicated. However, the key to understanding this is to realize that the methods of persuasive reasoning can surely work against us as much as they can work for us. Just as we have shoes to protect us from nature's briars we need certain reasoning techniques to protect us from suicidal food intake.

By now we trust that you have accepted the idea that eating the amount of food that is right for your height is also right for you. We also trust that you have accepted that the calories that you take in must contain the proper proportion of PROT, CHO, and FAT. There is more science to learn and apply as we go along but ERFYH boils down to these two factors: calories and content. That is it. There are only two factors to deal with and we must establish the behaviors that bring them to us. We must reason and we must behave in ways that are consistent with what we know about the human condition.

You for yourself

Now the task is to learn how to avoid faulty reasoning regarding your food intake by doing what CBT experts Tim Beck and Jesse Wright have termed becoming your own personal scientist.[52] With ERFYH we have established clearly that the program we recommend is you for yourself as opposed to you against yourself. Those of us who have spent years fighting ourselves as we faced overweight and obesity can certainly appreciate the difference in approach that is involved here. What we have called you for yourself uses the tools from good science that are the basis for CBT.

Let's get started with learning about CBT. We hope you will come to view CBT as a life saver. Picture CBT as one of those circles of kapok with several ropes on the side that you can grab onto and survive.

The "think system" that supports ERFYH

Let's return briefly to the musical from which we have borrowed the idea of a "think system" that can help us to accomplish ERFYH. What Professor Harold Hill did was to capitalize on a fundamental characteristic of human reasoning. It is unfortunate that he used it in a deceptive way to take money from some gullible Iowans. We will use it to be helpful. We will use the powers of our mind to overcome beliefs and behaviors that cause us to work against ourselves with regard to nutrition.

Dr. Joel Elkes[53] was very helpful to us when he told us that "mind is what the brain does." That simply means that we can take as a given that the brain can function in a way that is good for the body and therefore good for the brain. Mind and body are together when we are functioning normally. They are pitted against each other only when we choose to have it that way or when some form of disease causes it to happen. We can make choices. Those among us who are overweight or obese have made that sort of choice even though they may not have been aware of doing it when they did.

Cognitive behavioral theory is the scientific name for what we have referred to as the "think system." This theory holds that we cope with the "blooming, buzzing confusion" that we are born into. We do that by developing a unique set of automatic thoughts and schema. These two mental mechanisms usually make our coping more effective. It is possible for them to go wrong. Automatic thoughts can be inappropriately negative and generate negative feelings when more realistic automatic thoughts would not do so. When collections of automatic thoughts become systemized rather than associated with a single event or stimulus it is possible that our reasoning about an entire class of facts will become faulty. It is possible to develop a system of automatic thoughts known as a schema that applies to food generally instead of to specific foods. There are many ways that this could work against us. Viewing foods accurately is much more adaptive.

Suppose that one is in training to survive in very primitive environments such as those that military Special Forces have to face. The need for macronutrients and micronutrients is not altered just because the environment has changed. We can see how refusing to regard insects and snakes as appropriate food in that environment could be fatal. Making noise and risking discovery to acquire more conventional protein such as a pig might well be fatal. The attitude that one has toward food could well be the difference between living and dying.

It is much the same way with other attitudes toward food. If food becomes viewed as a source of comfort rather than a source of nutrition it will not be functioning as it should. Many more calories of the wrong content might be taken in as the individual attempts to meet an impossible goal. We might call the behavioral result of this schema eating to feel good. Eating has many purposes and is obviously necessary but there is a place for intelligent use of food. We have heard it said that wrenches make very poor hammers. The same reasoning applies to using food for something that it is not designed to do.

Applying the methods of science to ourselves is the way in ERFYH that we cope with automatic thoughts and schema that have us working against ourselves. Let's assume that we determine that we actually have developed the view that we are eating to feel good. What do we do?

We may begin monitoring or writing down the thoughts that come to us as we consider eating a meal or snack. What is it that we expect the intake of food to do for us? Is what we expect something that is reasonable for food to do? A simple way to accomplish this and preserve the record that we make has been called the double column technique. Its purpose is to evaluate our thoughts by recording them as either proper or improper. Once this task has been completed and with our thoughts out where we can consider them, we can decide whether we want to continue this thought pattern. We can make a decision that we are capable of making.

Suppose that we decide that we do not want this automatic thought to continue. Does our life experience teach us that just not wanting a thought will cause it to go away? Hardly! What we need is a method for dealing with the problem effectively. Fortunately, CBT provides us with just that sort of technique.

What we can do is develop a thought that is incompatible with what we might call the dysfunctional automatic thought. That could be something like: "I am eating because eating is necessary for life." When the idea of food comes up we then substitute the good thought for the bad thought. Is this easy? Of course it is not easy. Very few worthwhile efforts to change habits or dysfunctional thoughts are easy. The important thing for us to understand is that it is possible and that it becomes easier with practice. As we work through our library of dysfunctional automatic thoughts and schema we will find ourselves faced with easier and easier tasks.

French author and moralist Francois de La Rochefoucauld[54] described the way that we use CBT to achieve ERFYH. He said: "To eat is a necessity, but to eat intelligently is an art." CBT is about eating intelligently. It is also about a think system meaning that we use our mind to accomplish what we want to accomplish. Knowing that the mind works to use innate capacities uniquely to develop automatic thoughts and schema is just what we need in order to free us to eat intelligently. We are not prisoners of reflexes as frogs are. We are not locked into behavior that can never change. Nor are we limited to one environment.

Altering attitudes

It will not surprise us if you read about CBT and its application and conclude that you have encountered something at least a little bit like this before. Probably you have encountered what was called attitude. It is likely that the attitudes were being labeled as good or bad. "Have a good attitude" someone may have said to you when you were a member of a team. A coach might have said to your team "it's all about attitude." Your response might have been "what does attitude have to do with hitting a ball with the sweet spot of a baseball bat?"

Actually, CBT goes quite a bit farther with the concept of attitude and ties it to the other critical concepts that we have just discussed (automatic thoughts and schema). Here is the way we use this in ERFYH. We define attitude in a very specific way.

Attitude is a learned and specific predisposed way to respond to a specific set of stimuli.

Note that attitude is learned. It is learned according to the known laws of learning. Because it is learned it can be modified or unlearned. Once again it becomes clear that attitudes are not prison cells for which the key has been thrown away. Frogs may have fixed, unmodifiable responses but human beings have responses that can be modified.

In CBT it is helpful to look at the anatomy of attitudes. How are they constructed? There is a useful way of thinking that we will consider right now. Remember that the purpose of what we are doing is based on the fact that we are using the "think system" adapted from Professor Hill in learning to ERFYH. We are going to learn to eat intelligently.

Attitude is a function of	The Cognitive Component	The Perceptual Component
	The Motivational Component	The Affective Component

Or, put another way:

Attitude is a function of	What the individual KNOWS about the stimulus	How the individual SEES the stimulus
	What the individual WANTS from the stimulus	How the individual FEELS about the stimulus

Stimulus is used as a general term for any environmental event that presents itself to an individual as a whole or as a part. Stimulus may be general or specific. It may refer to Man or to a man.

We can add one more thing. Each component of the anatomy of an attitude interacts with every other component in all of the possible combinations. This may be illustrated in the following diagram:

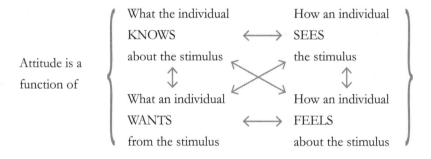

The principle is that everything affects everything else. Attitudes are mental but function as a system much as we view the human body as a system that is composed of many lesser systems all of which interact in some known or as yet unknown way.

We have found that many of those that we have tried to explain this to in the past let out a loud gasp when we came to this point. It can look like a mess. CBT actually has just given us a gift that will vastly simplify what we need to accomplish. If everything affects everything else it is not at all necessary for us to understand completely every component of a given attitude before we can do anything constructive. We can focus on what we can understand, modify it using CBT techniques, and be confident that the component that we do not fully understand will be modified also. It may even be modified in exactly the way we want.

Too complicated still? Let's take an example. Suppose we are talking about an attitude toward non-poisonous snakes. This is a good example because at one time we did extensive research on snake phobias that were disabling professionals. One of these professionals was an elementary school teacher who lived in fear that some boys would learn about her fear of snakes and smuggle a snake into the classroom. She was sure that if this happened she would experience terror, bolt from her classroom, and never again have control of the class. She felt that her whole career hinged on being able to overcome her fear of harmless snakes. That is why she came to us for help.

Despite our investigations we could not figure out what she might want from the feared stimulus, the snake. Therefore we focused mostly on altering what she actually knew about harmless snakes. We discovered that she inaccurately believed that snakes were very fast, slimy, aggressive, and likely to chase her if she ever confronted one of them. This was countered by changing what she knew. By observing harmless snakes from a safe place she was taught that snakes are relatively slow moving, have a great deal of difficulty in moving precisely on slick surfaces (such as the hardwood floors of a classroom), are scaly and not slimy, use escape (slithering away) if possible to get out of a situation that threatens them, and would run away from her rather than chase her.

This part of our attitude change effort had to be handled very skillfully. Not all snakes are harmless or slow. The Black Mamba of Africa is not only extremely aggressive and poisonous but is very fast moving over the ground and strikes very rapidly and often as it moves. It can travel as much as 14 mph and can strike hard and fast when threatened or when after prey. It is well documented that a single Black Mamba killed a 7,500 pound elephant. We emphasize that it is very much contraindicated to attempt persuading a person who is snake phobic with incorrect information. Snake phobic persons are known to be extremely adept at obtaining information about snakes and will rapidly detect misinformation that is provided to them. Loss of trust based on perceived attempts at manipulation can result in termination of therapy and probably fixation at the phobic level. Just as with ERFYH therapists must be certain that the information they are providing is absolutely accurate. Otherwise a simple "I don't know" and the suggestion to "find this out together" is appropriate. In CBT falling back on the idea of being one's own personal therapist is almost always a wise choice.

A critical problem was changing the teacher's perception of snakes as slimy. To do that we persuaded the teacher to touch a harmless snake that was being held by an assistant that she trusted. There was no way to sustain the belief that snakes were "slimy" after she conducted her own experiment (touching the snake). However, it was necessary to allow this perception to mature over some time. Immediately after touching the snake the teacher said "I know the snake is not slimy but that is still the way at I look at them for now. I will have to touch a lot of snakes before my attitude will be entirely different." Therapists have to be patient and allow cognitions to change in their own way according to our experience.

Our puzzlement about what the teacher wanted from not being afraid of a harmless snake was resolved in a surprising way. Over time we learned that she had developed a schema about snakes that was organized around the concept of control. She had come to believe that if she could overcome her fear of snakes she would be able to deal with almost anything that she might encounter in the classroom. What she wanted was to feel mastery. The schema which emerged well into the teacher's treatment by CBT had to do with a lot more than a fear of snakes. This was not at all apparent when we started the treatment. One can be sure that there will be a number of long forgotten automatic thoughts and schema that will surface as one moves toward ERFYH. The important thing will have been to have established skill in CBT that can be used as these automatic thoughts and schema emerge.

In assessing progress in CBT it is critical that we always defer the idea that there has been progress until we see clearly that the person's behavior and not just their talk has changed. There is an adage among experienced CBT practitioners: the muscles long remember what the mind has forgotten. In the treatment of alcoholism and other chemical addictions by CBT there is another adage: Watch the feet. The feet always tell the truth. We have applied this concept in Section 1 by saying that the bathroom scales are the best calorie counters. It is important that individuals understand ERFYH but it is much more important that the goals of ERFYH be met.

It will be obvious from looking at the models of attitude given above that the interaction of attitude components is a very powerful aspect of CBT. In this case what the teacher knew affected how she felt. How she felt affected how she saw the classroom situation generally and snakes specifically. The way she saw the situation affected what she discovered that she actually wanted in the situation. It all worked together.

Applying "attitude changes" to ERFYH

In this book we are addressing ERFYH not fear of snakes. We must not become distracted. One way to do that is to re-emphasize that the approach we are taking is anchored in solid science as well as practical experience. The late psychiatrist, Joseph Wolpe, in his seminal book *Psychotherapy by Reciprocal Inhibition,*[55] pointed out that human behavior changes for one of three reasons: maturation, lesions, and learning. The term lesions was used generally and referred to all forms of physical change in an individual's central nervous system due to trauma or psychoactive substances. Wolpe attributed the vast majority of behavior change in adults to learning. CBT is based in learning theory. It can be seen from this that we have in our hands the most powerful science that is available.

ERFYH is about learning to eat intelligently. It is also about using our mind or what our brain does in order to do what needs to be done to counter overweight and obesity and to mitigate atherosclerosis. Our starting place is with attitude which is defined as a learned and specific predisposed way to respond to a specific set of stimuli.

A way to do it

We will begin quite arbitrarily with the concept of "right" as in "eat right for your height." Please use the form in Appendix B to do the following exercise. Let your mind act without constraint and begin to record your thoughts about what you know about the concept of "right." Then do the same thing for what you think of about how you see (or perceive) "right." Next do the same thing for what you want and how you feel about the concept of "right." If you do this honestly and without constraints you may be quite surprised to find how it comes out.

Your first thought about "right" may be "something that is correct." But you may also have the thought "something I am entitled to have." Staying with what you know you may also say "being right has always been difficult for me." At this stage it does not matter at all what your thoughts may be: just write them down.

Do the same thing for the rest of the components of attitude using the handy form. Under what you want from "right," you may say "I think I want to do the right thing for myself and my family." You may say anything else. Just finish with the other components.

When you have finished recording your thoughts that are related to each of the components you will have taken a very, very crucial step. You will have taken the first step toward being what we term your own personal scientist. You will have collected and recorded data. Your collection will not be of opinion but of data. There can be no disputing that these are your thoughts or that they apply to you. There is a reason that the words are there. They reflect your thoughts about how you respond to the component, right, in ERFYH. The results may or may not have surprised you.

Explore this thinking. See where it takes you. It is possible that you will discover that your automatic thoughts about our suggestion that you eat "right" for your height are not only complex but may even provide a key to the reasons that you did not comply with diets that you tried in the past. "Right" may have been associated with restriction or loss of freedom. Trying to be "right" may have seemed desirable in order to reach a goal but it may also have meant having to knuckle under to some authority or some unpleasant reality.

Was it knuckling under to the "law" that one must control the amount of food that one takes in if he or she is going to achieve the weight that is correct for one's height that was doing you in? One individual put it this way: "I know what I have to do because of my height but I hate it. I have always hated being short and this is just one more thing that is bad about being short. Why is there this law?" Until the tool of being one's own personal scientist was available to this individual he had never realized how much he resented and opposed this restriction on his eating.

Decisions about automatic thoughts

With the fact that ERFYH includes becoming one's own personal scientist firmly established we are ready to go on. We may examine each of the automatic thoughts that we have written down. We must examine them in a very specific way. We list the pros and cons of keeping each thought as it is. In other words, what are the consequences of keeping our automatic thoughts just as they are? What is good about doing that and what is bad about doing that? Be brutally honest. It is possible that you will have to admit that you want to keep a ready source of irrational resentment. Acknowledge this and decide to pay the price for doing that if it is so.

Here is where the wisdom of many behavior change programs including the venerable Alcoholics Anonymous (AA)[56] come into play. To achieve behavior change there is no substitute for being rigorously honest with yourself. We and AA emphasize unequivocally that the honesty must be with one's self. Telling the truth to others but hiding it from one's self is the inevitable path to failure in ERFYH. It is far better to admit up front "I am just not going to do this" than to pretend. The reason? The latter behavior produces extreme chronic discomfort. Self hatred, depression, and a chronic feeling of failure will always accompany being dishonest with one's self. AA has had years of observing this and almost anyone who is overweight or obese is going to confirm that the consequences of being dishonest with one's self are horrible.

Let's say it again. If the truth is that the individual does not want what ERFYH has to offer it is important to say that up front. There are other ways to live life. It is far healthier to live in one of those ways than to fail again and again with ERFYH! Make no mistake about that. On the other hand, this book has advocated for a style of life that is based on ERFYH. We would not have done this if there were not a very real chance of success not only in overcoming overweight and obesity but also in mitigating atherosclerosis. Doing these things will open up a way of life that those who have it will never give up.

Back to the saddle

Suppose that you decide you want to change any automatic thought. This means that it will be necessary to propose some possible ways to do that. Think of several ways and then pick one. With that done you are ready to take the next step in becoming your own personal scientist. Set up an experiment to test whether your change technique has worked. After recording your starting point, indicating the date and the decision that was made, use the change technique for at least two weeks. Why two weeks? It is because our clinical experience indicates that automatic thoughts which don't change as soon as they are evident require at least two weeks to do what is called "extinguish." "Extinguish" is the scholarly term from the field of learning theory for disappear.

Here is an example using the idea that one does not like being at the mercy of one's height. When limiting the number of calories being taken in at a meal repeat the following: "I am not doing this because anyone is making me do it. I am doing it because I want to do ERFYH. I want the benefits of ERFYH for myself." Repeat this statement as many times as it is necessary to quell the feeling of resentment. Be certain that that has been accomplished. Don't stop too soon. This procedure is based in the clear scientific evidence that is available in what we regard as a subfield of CBT known as self-efficacy. It works.

At the end of two weeks or the end of whatever experimental period you choose record your thoughts about "right" once more. Use a ten point scale this time to assess the strength of your belief about the thought. Has it increased in strength, stayed the same, or decreased? If there has been change at all in the direction of decreasing the strength of the belief continue to use your device of silently talking to yourself when you face a situation that requires control. After a while you will find that your controlling behavior will continue but you will not be talking to yourself in the same way. Why? We don't know. However we do know that mind seems to work that way.

Continue this procedure with every automatic thought from every component of attitude. As you do this you will find that it becomes easier and quicker. It will become a way of life. We can promise you that. Be thorough at the very beginning and the results will come. Be sloppy at the beginning and we can promise you that the technique will not work. Mind is the part of our body that we are relying on and mind is like that for some reason.

A stop along the way

What has been accomplished thus far? First and almost without recognizing it you have decided to use ERFYH to meet your personal goal of dealing with overweight or obesity and mitigating atherosclerosis. The second thing is that you have accepted that you will proceed intelligently while using a most spectacular portion of your body known as the mind. You have learned that mind copes with the puzzling environment that it is born into by developing automatic thoughts and schema. These two entities drive behavior but they can be changed. In the third place you have applied the method of assessing automatic thoughts to the components of attitude. You have followed the method of being your own personal scientist and you have learned for yourself that it works. You have changed important automatic thoughts that you wanted to change and you have kept the automatic thoughts that you wanted to keep. You have accepted the consequences of doing either. The most important thing is that you have understood from your own efforts that you have a tool with which you can work. There is a saying that goes: It works if you work it.

How do we know?

It is mostly because we have been there. Each of us lived the life that many thought was normal as we grew up and we have suffered the kind of weight gain and atherosclerosis that goes with it. There were slight changes in the food industry that did not seem important to us. The initial use of margarine to replace butter is an example of this. We recall that many thought margarine was healthier than butter. We were unaware of what we were doing. That may not seem possible but it is true. We did not detect that our situation had changed from the relatively healthy habits of our youth to something else. We believed that the way we were eating was much like it had always been except for some enhancement that the food industry's nutritionists had discovered. We were puzzled when we seemed to be applying current knowledge but were drifting off course.

Now we know that we were up against changes in the food industry that we neither knew about nor understood. We read and studied and read and studied but the answers did not come for quite a while. By the time they did come we were so far off course that we felt lost. Then we discovered ERFYH. We added that to CBT. It was a long journey. For us it is not one that we can begin again. Harm has been done to us and we know it. But now we can share what we have learned with confidence. We know that you will be successful from this part of your journey on if you follow all aspects of ERFYH.

Elsewhere in this book we will address other aspects of ERFYH including methods for combating sugar addiction and using exercise properly as specific tools for ERFYH. We will offer some insights that we have had and we will encourage you to come up with your own. We know that you will become far more expert on your own form of ERFYH than we can ever be.

As teachers for most of our lives we will want most of all for you to know what we know but not because we taught it. We want you to know the truths about ERFYH for the simple reason that you discovered them for yourself. We want you to know from your own thought process and experience.

Final thoughts from others

Auto magnate Henry Ford shared some wisdom from his own life that we want to pass on. He said:

"Whether you think you can, or think you can't, you are right."

As we noted at the outset of this chapter Francois de La Rochefoucauld [French author and moralist (1613 - 1680)] put it this way:

"To eat is a necessity, but to eat intelligently is an art."

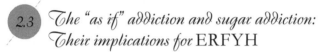

2.3 *The "as if" addiction and sugar addiction: Their implications for* ERFYH

What a word addiction is! It seems that every day we hear of a new "addiction." Coining a new adjective to add to addiction is almost becoming a popular sport. If one watches more television than is thought to be normal he is "addicted to television" or addicted to a particular program. The person is a (name the program) "junkie." Or it may be about using the internet or a phone. Someone is called a "Facebook" junkie or a "Twitter" junkie. It is very difficult to find anything precise or useful about this way of using the term.

It must be said also that there is a great deal of use for thinking of things as being much like a true addiction or even something that logically could be an addiction. It is this reason that keeps us from just scrapping the term and using something else. When we say that in becoming skilled at ERFYH one may have difficulty with an "as if" addiction to food we are using the concept in a helpful way. That is the purpose of having this chapter on addictions in Section 2. We are hopeful that this will be of use to you.

Understanding addiction

Many volumes have been written about addiction. There are many arguments about what constitutes an addiction and what does not. The interested reader will have no difficulty in finding his or her way into the various definitions, controversies, and the like. We have been there during our careers and can certify that the study of this area will be very interesting. Our purpose in this book will not be served by an attempt to synthesize all of the relevant data and theories about addiction. Instead we offer our own view of what is most important for ERFYH.

We begin by noting that the word addiction is rooted in a concept from ancient law that provided for a person to become slave-like if he failed to pay debts. An officer of the court could rule that the person had lost his or her civil rights and had become unable to exercise the power to will his own activity. In effect, the person's will power was rendered inoperative.

It is not much of a logical jump to go from appearing to lack will power due to a decision of the court to losing the power to exercise one's will due to some substance. The addicted person seems not to have the power to say "no" to the substance to which he is addicted. The addicted person may promise many times to stop using heroin, cocaine, or alcohol but be simply unable to keep the promise.

There are many theories of alcoholism and other addictions that have generated a myriad of studies of varying quality and utility. Each seems to illuminate some of the phenomena and obscure others. There is no single, integrative theory that we can adopt for this chapter. Therefore, we are going to base our discussion in the most tried and true of ideas about addiction to alcohol and its treatment. Alcoholics Anonmymous was founded as an approach to alcoholism but its underlying theory and famous "12 steps" have been adopted widely as the basis for understanding and treating addiction to other substances including narcotics. Students have been able to trace the principles of many behavior change procedures to AA as well as to the phenomenon of conversion. While time, experience, and research have revealed inconsistencies and errors in what the founders of AA began with over fifty years ago, millions of individuals who have been addicted to alcohol have found a way to overcome the addiction. They have used what AA suggested as a program of recovery. We do not hesitate to borrow concepts from AA or any other method of behavior change if doing so will enhance the chance of ERFYH. Our view is that "what works, works."

At the core of AA's traditions is the idea that addiction consists of two components. The components are an allergy and an obsession. These are regarded as inseparable. They are always found together just as we know from Section 1 that glucose and fructose are found together in nature. Science has discovered a great deal more about these two components since the founding of AA. These days we use the term allergy as a convenient fiction when what we really mean is psychopharmacological effect. The latter simply means that when we introduce a foreign substance into the brain it usually results in a change in behavior. Such changes in behavior can be quite dramatic.

Perhaps the most sensational demonstration of this effect occurred when a construction worker, Phineas Gage, was present during a tunnel excavation accident. There was an explosion and a drilling tool was propelled into Gage's head. Usually this meant immediate death but Gage survived. Gage lived for many years thereafter. Throughout his lifetime Gage's behavior certainly changed. It was serendipitous that he survived because his condition allowed science to learn a great deal about brain-behavior relationships that are expressed as what we know as personality.

Much less dramatic and life threatening methods of introducing foreign substances into the brain are quite common. We can mention drinking alcohol, snorting cocaine, smoking marijuana, and the like. We find the principle is the same. If we introduce certain substances into the brain by whatever means we can predict changes in a wide range of behavior, emotion, and cognition. The field of psychopharmacology is defined by the study of these phenomena.

Most all of us have seen the equivalent of what Gage experienced when a foreign substance such as an anesthetic has been introduced into a brain for medical purposes. Not everyone accepts the idea of certainty or inevitability. The myth persists that it is possible for human beings to use will power to overcome the effect of the substance. We know from personal experience that under anesthesia all sorts of things can be done to an individual and he will do nothing to stop it because the effect of an anesthetic is biochemical and beyond our control. That does not prevent our hearing statements such as "I drive better after a few beers because I am not so tense" or "drugs like cocaine just don't affect some people." Every addiction specialist has heard these things said many times. These false beliefs are very strongly held. Even worse is the fact that individuals are expected to sober up quickly in the face of an emergency or other demand. We hear the statement frequently from spouses that he or she "could stop drinking if they loved me." The addict's continued use of alcohol or heroin is viewed as evidence of lack of love rather than a simple physical fact. This greatly complicates treatment.

Fundamentals of treating addiction

The oldest and most successful program for dealing with alcoholism requires as its first step that the alcoholic make an admission. That admission is of the form: "We admitted that we were powerless over alcohol, that our lives had become unmanageable." Addiction treatment professionals understand that without this admission treatment is almost never successful.

Several things stand out when we look at this first step. The first is the idea that one has become powerless over a substance. Technically the powerlessness is only over that substance after it is ingested. Cases and cases of liquor may remain on store shelves and be of no consequence to the alcoholic. Yet putting even a very small amount into the body can lead to the second important aspect of addiction that we must understand. Life for the addicted person has become unmanageable. It is not just that the body is being attacked by a toxin and that organs are being damaged. It is that the person's entire life is in chaos. Mental impairment will have become profound. Shortly after the addictive substance has been eliminated from the addict's body it may be assumed that he or she will be the old self again. Nothing could be further from the truth and the failure to understand this undeniable fact accounts for a great deal of the misery associated with addiction. The addicted individual and all members of the problem pay dearly for this misunderstanding.

Our clinical experience has clearly shown that alcoholism requires approximately 9 to 15 months of abstinence before the physical effects of alcohol dissipate to the degree that they will dissipate. Until that period has passed it is best if the addict, law enforcement representatives or regulators, employers, and all other members of the problem consider the individual to be under the influence to some degree. We believe that two to five years of abstinence are required for the alcoholic to develop a lifestyle that does not require alcohol. We do not know whether other addictions follow the same time table. But it is prudent for the therapist and all other members of the problem to work with these timetables in mind. There is no reason at all to suspect that the timetables will not apply to so called food addiction that we mention later.

During the first years of the addiction recovery process one can assume that the addicted person will become increasingly aware of past levels of impairment. The alcoholic who remains abstinent will experience growing awareness that he became a staggering inebriate. It will be recognized that muscle coordination, cognition, and speech became profoundly affected. It is not only the addicted who fail to perceive cognitive and physical impairment. Normal experimental subjects who are at legal blood alcohol levels can tell that they are not driving well but they remain unable to do what is needed to correct their behavior. Introduction of a foreign substance has changed brain function whether we intended it or did not.

There are both general and idiosyncratic effects of impairment. One individual may suffer severe speech impairment while another may simply go to sleep. Intake of alcohol always triggers a degree of physical impairment which AA termed an allergy. It also produces a psychological effect which AA called an obsession. More complicated terms and qualifications may be used in light of more recent knowledge but we hold here that the fundamental lesson is what counts. Foreign substances that are introduced into the brain have a combination of physical and psychological effects that have to be dealt with.

It is much less clear whether addiction can exist in the absence of a known addictive substance. Is it possible for ordinary foods to have addictive properties? We know that foods that are commonly eaten by the majority of human beings can be toxic to a few. The term food allergy is used to describe this phenomenon. Barrett and Drogin[57] have coined the term addictions without substance to describe so called behavioral addictions such as gambling addiction and sex addiction. We are using another concept to describe something that appears to be an addiction without the presence of a known addictive substance. We call this the "as if" addiction.

The "as if" addiction

It is often said that if it walks like a duck and quacks like a duck it surely is a duck. Experience tells us that this is not always so. It is a common experience to learn that what one thought was so was not so. If nothing else persuades us that we cannot always believe our own eyes exposure to an expert illusionist will do it. Does anyone really believe that the eyes shown in a painting actually move as one walks from one side of a room to the other? Nobody believes such a thing but observers will insist that the eyes in some paintings appear to follow them.

A logical trap for the person who is attempting to assess addiction of any kind is the assumption that the assessor knows the history of the individual who is being observed. The drinking of alcohol or the use of drugs may have been observed or assumed to have happened based on some information. That does not mean that the observed behavior is actually due to having put a psychoactive substance into the brain. We must accept that there may have been no such event.

The famous learning theorist, Burros F. Skinner, taught us that behavior that was under some kinds of reinforcement control could look very much like addiction.[58] His device to illustrate what he meant was a specially constructed box that permitted him to monitor the behavior of an animal and dispense a reward such as a food pellet when the animal exhibited the behavior that was desired. Skinner discovered that an animal's behavior changed markedly according to the way the animal received his rewards. Giving a reward every time the behavior occurred resulted in very fast learning but the behavior stopped very quickly if Skinner stopped providing the reinforcement. If he established the behavior instead by giving a pellet on the third or later time that the behavior was observed the learning occurred more slowly but it lasted longer once the reinforcement was withdrawn. A third schedule of reinforcement varied the ratio of behaviors to reinforcement, the interval between reinforcements, and the connection to the animal's next behavior. In that case the experimenter could provide the reward or reinforcement according to a predetermined ratio of something like 1:3 and also according to a variable interval such as every 30 seconds. Under this schedule of reinforcement the pellet reward was given only if there was another occurrence of the desired behavior. Looking at this situation as a human being might we can say that the situation was about as uncertain as it could get. Just what were the rules that governed the situation? How does one determine those rules? The important practical aspect of this manipulation of reward is that the target behavior endured very long after the experimenter had stopped the reinforcement altogether.

There is another practical consequence of this sort of reinforcement schedule. An observer who did not know about what the experimenter had been up to might look at the target behavior and conclude that it was just natural. There would be no evidence that the behavior had been manipulated by a reward or what psychologists call reinforcement of a target behavior. The observer might well think that the animal had become addicted to a substance that had no known addictive quality. It would appear that there was addiction to the substance when it was actually the unknown pattern of reinforcement that was accounting for the behavior. It can be that food has reinforcing characteristics for human beings while looking as if it has addictive qualities.

We can complicate this a bit more. It has become known that simply doing something will make it more likely to be done again. Experimental Psychologists have discovered that an action reinforces that very action. This is what is behind the strategy that we describe in our chapter on exercise when indicating what to do until motivation comes. Acting "as if" you want to do ten minutes on the treadmill will lead to wanting to do ten minutes on the treadmill. Every person who has ever tried to begin a regimen of working out knows this from personal experience. They know equally well that not doing what has been scheduled makes it much more difficult to do what has been scheduled the next time. These are experiences we can count on. ERFYH advises that they be used.

We can see at this point that addiction involves an experience that is much like slavery. One's power to decide has been taken away somehow. This may be due to a chemical that acts directly on the brain and therefore on the mind or it may be due to an unfortunate or unintentional history of reinforcement. It is very natural and adaptive for the human being to learn. That is the way that infants bring order out of the blooming buzzing confusion referred to by William James.[59] It is also natural for the human being to learn things that there was no intent to learn. The latter is called incidental one trial learning. Examples of one trial learning are legion and we will leave it up to the reader to look to personal experience for examples. It will be an instructive experience to do so.

There is no better example of an "as if" addiction than what has been called food addiction. It is clearly possible that some foods have addictive qualities. Certain foods may have quite specific effects on certain areas of the mammalian brain as well. There are so called hedonic pathways that have been identified in the brains of experimental animals. Human beings have reported phenomena after eating certain foods which seem to be very much like those associated with substances that are known to have addictive properties. Discussion of this literature is beyond the scope of his book. We simply take this as a given.

What we can do is to suggest that behaviors that are very much like addictive behaviors can be observed in those who are overweight or obese. This understanding can be helpful when we ask why people don't just do ERFYH as soon as they find out what the science behind it is. The explanation may be that they no longer own their own will power due to some chemical that they have ingested. It may be something else. It could well be that the behavior is under simple or complicated reinforcement control. We know that those who are addicted to cocaine report that intense craving can be triggered by the single passage in a song that was listened to as part of the addiction experience. It is just as possible that the trigger for food binging could be part of a song or other event.

With ERFYH we are fortunate that it does not matter whether an addictive food exists or whether the individual is under some form of reinforcement control that the therapist or observer can't define. The remedial processes are the same. They include processes from AA, the unlearning or extinction literature, and those from CBT.

It is necessary to amplify our earlier remarks about the nature of what we are calling food addiction. Mostly this amplification has to do with understanding the severity of the addiction. The issue of severity of impairment is very often overlooked when overweight or obesity is involved. The person who acts "as if" they are without will power is not likely to be cognitively impaired. There is no stuttering or stammering. There is no staggering or falling. The person does not lose consciousness. They do not smell of spirits. They are just carrying too much fat. Nothing more need be said.

This view is very much mistaken. Overweight and obesity in addition to causing the physical problems that we outlined in Section 1 also cause massive interference with one's life. Anyone who has been overweight or obese can verify what we have just said. It is hard to think of any activity requiring mobility that will not be affected by excess weight. What would it be? Gardening? Just think of bending over to clean out weeds from tomato plants and running into one's own accumulated fat. Walking from one floor to another while doing housework? Think of carrying 25 excess pounds of FAT. It is no different from carrying 25 pounds of lead in a backpack as you walk up and down stairs. Shopping? Think of carrying excess weight as you walk from store to store looking for that just right pair of shoes. It is very safe to say that if an activity involves mobility overweight or obesity is interfering with it. Life is less manageable for the overweight and obese.

Our most recent example of this fact came when we were notifying a friend of another friend's being in a rehabilitation facility due to an illness. We knew that the friend we were notifying would be concerned and want to help her sick friend in some morale building way. When we called the friend she let us know that she had some mobility issues. As a grossly overweight person it was clear that our friend had developed knee and hip problems and had undergone joint replacement surgery. She was unable to do her usual caring actions when she definitely wanted to do them. Parking in the facility's parking lot and walking to the unit was beyond what she could do. Not being able to assist a friend turned out to be a cost of being obese. An honest assessment of obesity indicates that there is almost no physical activity that will not become enhanced if we do ERFYH successfully. Life can again become manageable. The overweight or obese person can rightly say that life has become unmanageable just as an alcoholic might say that.

We have been very frustrated in times gone by as we have attempted to explain ERFYH. At about this point of our explanation individuals seem to glaze over and we begin to lose them. Perhaps this is because we are making the point much too complicated. We can simplify by stating that it is possible for food to have reinforcing properties but not addictive properties. Any substance, activity, or thought that strengthens a behavior that it is associated with is said to have reinforcing properties. It is a matter of definition on the basis of an empirical observation. We know that food pellets strengthen the association between a stimulus event and a behavior. This has been demonstrated reliably using experimental rats. Food pellets are reinforcers by definition. That does not mean that food pellets are addictive.

Some may believe that we are rearguing the traditional mind-body dichotomy here. That is not at all true. Our position was stated earlier when we cited Dr. Joel Elkes. This world famous psychiatrist provided the perspective that medicine has long recognized. Mind is what the brain does. For convenience of exposition of our ideas we are dividing the physical and psychological while specifying that there is no separation between mind and body.

Addiction to sugar

It may appear that we have left the concept of food addiction behind us. We have not done that. There is one class of substances that is a major candidate for being an addictive food rather than a reinforcement. Yet there is a paradox. The substance occurs in nature and in that form it is not addictive. It is only when man acts on this natural substance and concentrates it that it becomes so harmful or addictive.

Repeatedly in this book we have pointed out that man has adapted to the substances in his environment that provide the macronutrients: PROT, FAT and CHO. This is a process that has taken thousands or perhaps a couple of million years. We have also pointed out that one of these substances is readily available to man in its natural form. It is found in unprocessed fruit. Dry the fruit and make raisins and one has altered natural fruit into a more concentrated form of sugar that is unhealthy. Collecting sap from a maple tree and boiling it for a while generates maple syrup. Maple syrup is a very sweet and concentrated form of sugar.

We find that modern man must deal with the fact that table sugar (sucrose, 50% glucose and 50% fructose) is available almost exclusively in an unnatural, very concentrated form. We do not need to be apologetic in saying that there is not much to indicate that common natural foods are addictive but there still may be sugar addiction. The concept of sugar addiction is useful as one tries to deal with overweight and obesity. It must be made clear that any such addiction would almost certainly be due to the man-made or concentrated form of what is relatively harmless to most individuals. Imagine how many clumps of grapes one would have to eat in order to obtain the amount of sugar that is present in a cup of raisins. The human stomach would be bulging. We can also ask ourselves the number of apples that one would have to eat in order to obtain as much fructose as one might get from a small amount of high fructose corn syrup (HFCS) sweetened cereal. To be sure the stomach could be painfully full before the equivalent was reached.

It would be error for us to suggest that science has fully accepted the concept of sugar addiction. It has not. We can say that there is sufficient evidence to assume that further research will establish that fact. There are many new techniques for researchers to use and there are good groups that are pursuing this line of research. There is one more thing that makes us comfortable with asserting that sugar is addictive. The techniques for dealing with obstacles to ERFYH are the same regardless of whether sugar is or is not addictive. There is no doubt that it is wise to reduce the intake of HFCS and sucrose. Accepting that HFCS and sucrose are addictive substances and using the treatments that are known to help with addictions to reduce their ingestion will help anyone accomplish ERFYH.

We can find no harm in proceeding in that manner. Therefore, from this point on in this chapter we will refer to sugar addiction without further qualification. We will take this as a given.

The notion that sucrose or table sugar as derived from sugar beets and cane can be an addictive substance is neither new nor novel. A cursory search on the internet will reveal many references that have expounded on that topic over the years. Our perspective, however, is quite different. We emphasize that a food-like substance[60] that began to be manufactured a little over thirty years ago is very likely to be much more addictive than even the more concentrated forms of natural sugar that man has devised. Why is this? It is because HFCS is cheaper and in a liquid form to accommodate shipping. Manufacture of HFCS now expands the availability of two substances that are found in nature where they are in a much less concentrated form. HFCS is composed of 42-55% fructose and 45-58% glucose but commonly it is found to be 55% fructose and 45% glucose.

A diet that is limited to natural sources of sweetness such as glucose or fructose is not likely to be harmful. We have found no sources that suggest that the quantities of sugar that occur naturally in fruits or vegetables that have not been processed would ever be sufficient to precipitate much harm or addiction. Facts suggest that the human body is superbly adapted to the environment in which it has evolved. Unlike the New Zealand cave glow worms that we referred to earlier that are dependent on a specific environment we are able to adapt. Changing our environment is not likely to become disastrous all at once. Exceptions today are diabetes and atherosclerosis. There is an epidemic rate of diabetes growing amongst us and atherosclerosis is rampant in the U.S. and worldwide. It seems possible that the human being has met his match in coping with what is happening.

Adding the characteristic of addiction to the process greatly complicates the task of health care professionals. A straight forward process would permit healthcare professionals to advise those at risk to limit sugar intake to that from fruits and vegetables in order to keep the quality and quantity of food at the correct level (follow ERFYH). It would be done. When an addictive process is added to any system that aims to maximize quality of life through dietary changes it means the effort must do much more than advise about nutrition. It must deal with one of the most difficult diseases of mind that man has encountered.

Coping with sugar addiction

Let's get very personal. We have documented that the major dietary factor in driving the development of atherosclerosis, overweight, and obesity is fructose. We knew that it was absolutely necessary for the validity of this viewpoint to show that both the overweight and those of optimal weight are vulnerable to atherosclerosis. It was equally mandatory that we find an explanation of atherosclerosis that accounted for its occurrence in both the obese and those of appropriate weight. We met both of these requirements in Section 1. We trust that we did that to your satisfaction. If we did not accomplish our goal in Section 1, we recommend re-reading it.

At the beginning of the authors' journey of understanding together we asked ourselves how the so called Standard American Diet (SAD) accumulated so much fructose. We studied food labels and recipes but repeatedly missed the critical points because of two errors. The first error was in not realizing how creative the food industry has become in using synonyms for sucrose and HFCS on food labels. We found that there was far more sugar in food than was apparent at first impression. Our second error was in overlooking the fact that sweetness has become progressively more important in the SAD.

It is worth noting that slaves on plantations in Brazil and the Carribean Islands and in the U.S. who frequently chewed on sugar cane did not develop diabetes. It was the wealthier who could afford table sugar or concentrated sucrose who were more likely to develop disease. The overall risk was low at that time but today the risk is very high. There has been no change in the human body. The change has been environmental. There has become a demand for increasing sweetness that could not be met as it had been met in the past. A different and cost effective way had to be found to meet the demand. That way was found but the desire for sweetness is being met in a fashion that has dire consequences for an organism that is not ready for it. We are not far from the sort of major consequence that there would be for the New Zealand Cave Glow Worms if their environment had even a very tiny change.

Consumers are finding that HFCS availability has coincided with food labels that are becoming more and more difficult to interpret. Synonyms for HFCS have been developed and it has been possible to load many foods with sweetness that can't be attained naturally and thereby increase profits. Pollan[61] calls such foods "food-like substances." We were very confused by these changes for quite a while. It was easy to conclude that HFCS did not differ from fructose as it occurs in nature. It has taken some time for the difference between these two substances to be appreciated. We now know and now other consumers can know also.

The plight of the sugar addicted

Wise men have said throughout most of man's history that we should not criticize a person until we have walked a mile in his moccasins. Here we are compelled to state that no human experience makes this statement more meaningful than sugar addiction. It is certainly true that there are those who still do not take in a great deal of concentrated sucrose or HFCS and become addicted. These individuals nevertheless may ingest well more fructose than is necessary to create atherosclerosis. They will not have to face what the overweight and obese face day in and day out but they will face other health consequences.

Overweight and obese individuals face a dilemma. They are encouraged to lose weight for health and attractiveness reasons at the same time that the very food they are routinely induced into eating is laced with the very substance that that they must not have if they are to return to being healthy. It is the equivalent of force feeding alcohol into the alcoholic and then blaming him for being unable to avoid being intoxicated.

We could say that it is even worse. The alcoholic can never miss the fact that he or she is taking in alcohol. If the taste of alcohol is obscured by other substances the undeniable effects are still soon evident. Speech is slurred, staggering begins, and cognition is impaired. This is not the case for the individual who is addicted to sugar. This addicted person is very unlikely to detect exactly which substance is in the food or food-like substance that he or she has ingested. It is true that some individuals report a sugar high but for most people the effect of ingesting either a concentrated but natural substance or a manufactured substance will be long term rather than immediate.

Overweight, obesity, and atherosclerosis just do not happen overnight. One wag said that it is like watching corn grow. Over time it is obvious that a seed has become a corn stalk. Just when did it happen? Indeed, those who are neither overweight nor obese may believe that they are safe from atherosclerosis when the facts show that they too are quite vulnerable to the effects of fructose. This is a time of pervasive use of sucrose and HFCS and use of synonyms on food labels to disguise that fact. Consumers will have to expend great effort in order to avoid taking in this toxic substance. Imagine the furor that would occur if a tasteless form of pure alcohol were put into nearly every drink or food that we use. That is exactly what is happening to sugars. The vulnerable person will find it difficult to find a breakfast cereal that has not been laced with sucrose and HFCS. Some foods may report containing sugar in four different forms. Sucrose, corn syrup (glucose from corn starch), fructose syrup (about 90% fructose) and HFCS may be listed on the same label. The unwary consumer will not add up all of these sweeteners and assess accurately the amount of sugars that are being ingested.

There are many reasons to be more understanding of what the obese and overweight are facing today. It is well documented that food not contaminated by concentrated sucrose or HFCS is difficult to obtain from foods that are in the groceries that serve the most vulnerable. For the most part this is a function of economics. Michael Pollan[62] has taught us that food that our grandmothers would have recognized as food is much more expensive than the food-like substances that are found in the center aisles of food markets these days. The latter are not only cheaper to provide in the first place but they also have long shelf life. They do not rot. They also are associated with reduced time spent in the kitchen.

Pollan reports having had a common food-like substance on his desk for many years. It has not rotted and roaches will not eat it. Those are excellent reasons for us not to eat it.

Appreciating the difficulty that the afflicted have in dealing with obesity and overweight is not too difficult if we try our hand at it. Stores that stock food that our grandmothers would recognize as food are found typically in affluent neighborhoods. It costs money just to have access to these stores if one does not live in those neighborhoods. The cost of transportation to the store and back may make going there impossible. Once access has been gained the food even costs more! More trips to the grocery will need to be made because actual food will spoil and rot. Roaches and vermin will eat it if it is unprotected. Increased cost of fuel obviously works against the most conscientious of those in recovery from sweetness addiction. These factors lead the overweight and obese to become more overweight and obese as well as atherosclerotic. Decreased mobility, agility, and mood further degrade the ability to utilize anti-addiction treatments. Problems are compounded on top of problems. If we desire to change this situation in an individual's life we must first understand it. It has been said that one cannot fix a problem if he does not know he has it. Advertisers years ago warned us about bad breath that our best friends would not tell us that we had. Many forces are at work today to keep the full implications of overweight, obesity, and atherosclerosis from us. Clinicians and lay people need to become wiser.

The point to be taken away from what we have just said is that the increased use of the one taste enhancing substance that has changed substantively in the past 300 years or so is not only physically harmful but addictive in its very nature. We can truly express concern about salt, fat and sugar while emphasizing that the worst of these is sugar. That is what the thin and atherosclerotic and those who are overweight, obese, and addicted as well as atherosclerotic, are facing. It is an alarming picture. We need to be sympathetic in looking at the plight of the sugar addicted. It is fitting to say there but for the Grace of God go I.

It all started with a cookie

Let's listen to the story of an individual who faces sugar addiction. His story is the source of one of the sub-titles of this chapter.

Butch started watching his weight when he was a college freshman. He should have started much earlier because as a paper boy at age thirteen he routinely washed down a half dozen Danish pastries with a quart of milk after he finished his route. HFCS had not been developed at that time so he faced only calories from milk, flour, and sugar. Butch went home to have breakfast after finishing off the pastries and milk.

There were obese individuals in his family but Butch seemed to be able to eat without gaining weight until he went to college. Butch graduated from high school weighing 145 pounds. He quickly gained ten pounds in his first year of college and by the time he graduated from college he weighed 165. For many years, Butch struggled to maintain that weight by various means. He used exercise such as playing handball, running marathons, fasting, diets of numerous types, etc. His struggle was successful for many years but eventually it failed. By his late sixties, Butch weighed 220 pounds. None of the methods that he had used in the past for weight control were working and he always failed to lose weight. A medical event scared Butch straight. He lost fifty pounds and became relatively stable at 170 pounds. He was not able to lose enough weight to be right for his height but Butch had some positive results overall.

Butch also had problems with a mildly elevated fasting plasma glucose level. He restricted his sucrose intake to near zero and limited his deliberate intake of fructose to fruits and vegetables. He was declared not to be diabetic. His HgA1C test for five years routinely scored at about 5.5 which is below the cut-off score for T2DM.

When Butch went on a month's cruise he faced the usual elaborate buffets and dessert offerings that cruise ships pride themselves on offering. He had no problem avoiding desserts at the regular meals. One evening he and his wife found their way to the evening desserts that the ship made available after its stage shows. He had a cookie. Night after night the couple went back to the evening dessert offerings and soon they both were having ice cream and cookies routinely. Butch was puzzled. The more cookies he had the more he wanted!

This pattern of behavior is exactly like that of an alcoholic who has slipped (had just one drink). The behavior continued after the cruise when Butch returned home. He found himself returning to patterns of behavior that had plagued him in previous years. Butch was often out during the day at lunch time. He went to fast food restaurants although he knew that the foods there were loaded with HFCS. He found himself scheduling meetings around lunches and dinners. Butch thought he should be gaining weight but he was not. His weight remained steady. Butch weighed every day as required by ERFYH and there was very little change for a while. Then the weight gain started, the craving for sugar began, and within a few weeks he had gained a dozen pounds. Butch tried to counter this but soon found himself to be grazing. Grazing is the term used to describe almost constant intake of small amounts of sucrose or other nutrients. He avoided fruits and vegetables for the most part but when he had them the amounts increased. The coping skills that Butch had learned in ERFYH were no longer applied. Skills that enhanced sugar intake and weight gain grew stronger and more frequently used.

Butch realized that his sugar addiction had returned in full force. He returned to ERFYH procedures but found it very difficult to do so. He had gained almost twenty pounds and he found that his cognitions about weight monitoring were being neglected.

Butch's story is almost a classic description of relapse as it occurs in all addictions. The first small instance of non-compliance did not as he feared result in any huge negative consequences. He escalated. It appeared that he could violate the ERFYH procedures with impunity. He found more and more reasons to depart from a successful program of recovery. Butch became more and more disgusted with himself and increased his emotional eating as time went by. Today, we do not know whether Butch will be able to return to ERFYH. There is a saying in AA that applies very well in Butch's case: The saying goes: "I know I have another drunk in me: I don't know whether I have another recovery in me." Only time will tell for Butch.

Grazing: a serious obstacle to dealing with sugar addiction

Here is another aspect of the sugar addicted person's plight. Take as a given that a behavior known as grazing is a major obstacle to ERFYH. Add to that the fact that the objects of the grazing have changed their nature. The piece of cake containing 200 calories that one ate in 1970 has become super-sized and now contains perhaps 500 calories. Exactly the same behavior is now adding 300 more calories. The person who learned to graze years ago is dealing today with a substance that is addictive and does not know it.

If we look back toward our distant ancestors who were the hunter-gatherers we probably will find them to have been grazers. Finding and ingesting food was a full time job. When our ancestors found food they most likely ingested that food when and where they found it. There was just not enough food readily available all the time and our digestive system had to be ready to deal with food at any time it became available.

If we keep this history in mind it can be concluded that there is nothing harmful to us if we keep up a steady behavior of ingesting food. We can eat when we want to and our system will be able to handle it because it evolved a way to do just that. This is very good news to anyone who is attempting to deal with obesity. Eating can be fun. Food tastes good. Food is readily available. It would appear that there would be no harm in taking food in when and where we find it. That appearance is deceptive. By the time the addicted person is ready to confront the problem there can be harm in taking in food when and where we find it. There can be harm in grazing. Readers of Section 1 already know that ERFYH calls for three meals per day and perhaps a snack in the evening. The reasons for this are well documented in Section 1. It is not because the human body has changed in this blink of an evolutionary eye. It is because the environment has become more under man's control and he has changed the environment. The human body has had to adapt to another reality.

The reality is that today grazing is no longer difficult. Food can be found easily and in sufficient quantities at almost any time. With the onset of high calorie crops and domesticated food animals we face the situation of having food of all kinds readily available to us. Further, the food can be stored safely or preserved. That means that our natural grazing behavior can be turned against us. Instead of working hard for a small bite of food we find that we need only go to the refrigerator for a piece of cheese or to a kitchen cabinet to have some potato chips. It is easy. The source of our food is not in nature but in the grocery store or the fast food restaurant. This means that our digestive system can be put to work for many hours of a day on incredibly large amounts of food if we choose. There is no balance between the demands for energy use in hunting and gathering and the intake of energy. It is easy for us to take in far more food than we need. The food we take in need not be the kind of food that we used to find in natural settings. The food we take in need not be healthful even if it allows us to feel sated.

Let's add another factor. Our ancestors were faced only with food that could be found in nature. That food had certain characteristics and we developed an incredibly effective taste capacity that allowed us to recognize what was and what was not appropriate food. Our senses permitted us to detect unsafe food and to take in safe food. Spoiled food was unsafe and its smell was not difficult to detect. With the same senses today we face large quantities of food that will not spoil or otherwise become bad for us through natural processes. Milk is not only homogenized to keep fat in solution but it is pasteurized. Bacteria that would spoil it for us have been killed by heat. The sweet taste of high calorie foods is available to us now in many forms that were unknown in our species' earliest days. We can rely on refined sucrose, HFCS, and large engineered apples to bring us the sweet taste. What once struck our sense of taste as a slight tapping now hits it as a loud bass drum. That food is available to us at our whim in very large quantities. We don't even have to work for it.

Today's reality

We need to transition to a discussion that is more clearly related to the reality of today. It is true that we have a system that is well adapted to grazing but those who are obese need to pretend that it is not adapted to grazing. ERFYH needs one to assume a new reality. Our system is no longer superbly adapted to the kind of grazing that it formerly found productive. Grazing has to be severely limited. If we follow ERFYH and eliminate grazing we can realize the sort of appropriate weight that was common just a few decades ago. There has to be some way for us to inhibit the grazing habit. It is necessary to begin acting "as if" proper food is only available at certain times of our day and in relatively small amounts at that.

Here, it is necessary to review what we know about CBT and look at it with a slightly different perspective. We can begin with a basic truth. What we do and how we think about it governs how we feel. There is no doubt that this is fact. Most overweight or obese persons agree that it is better to feel good about their body instead of feeling bad about it. Not to be obese is preferred to being obese. We have to modify what we do and how we think about it in order to get there. What we need to do has been described above. Now we have to alter what we know or think about it.

The reader will recognize that this requires us to utilize what was learned above about attitude. We will accomplish this by looking at attitude from a slightly different perspective. We know from the outset that it will be composed of the cognitive (knowing) factor, the perceptual (seeing) factor, the motivational (wanting) factor, and the affective (feeling) factor.

Grazing or constantly looking for and ingesting food is natural to us. Our culture may have taught something different. We may have been taught to take meals three times per day. We can adapt to this although it is really against our nature to do it. There may be a great deal of elation when we discover the joy of taking in food any time the notion strikes us. Our behavior is taking us back to an earlier time. There remains the question of whether we can do both what is natural for us and what is good for us in our present environment.

The answer is yes provided that we can add to our CBT skills a technique known as "mental imagery". This technique allows us to create an environment that is specific to ourselves. We can imagine ourselves in a slightly modified situation where our ancestors may have been. We can be in an environment where we are required to look for food constantly but find it only occasionally. We can make that environment real just as we may invest ourselves in an acting role. The simplest way to start is to define finding food as finding mealtime. We can require that our grazing be unsuccessful for a while as it probably was often unsuccessful for our hunter-gatherer ancestors. When it is meal time we can say that our hunting and gathering has been successful. Using mental imagery we place ourselves so that we are again living in a place where food is scarce and we find it only every once in a while. The fact is that we find food only at meal times as defined by ERFYH.

When we find food in the environment that we are creating we make sure that it is only in the form of the macronutrients and micronutrients that we need. This means that we take in the correct amount of calories as PROT, the correct amount of calories as CHO, and the correct amount of calories as FAT. The macronutrients in this case can take any form that is found in nature. No processed or food-like substances are acceptable. The calories are limited as required in Section 1. Section 1 has provided also the way to determine the number of calories required to maintain one's desired weight. The hunter-gatherer that we have made of ourselves through mental imagery only finds that number of calories.

More specific methods of coping with sugar addiction

Sugar addiction is a problem. We continue to take that as a given because every known method of problem solving begins with defining the problem. Sugar addiction from this perspective is no different from any other problem that we might have to solve. We have to decide what the problem is before we can design a program for coping with it. That task is rather simple where sugar addiction is concerned. We have ingested a substance that is addictive and therefore both mind and body have been affected and probably afflicted. There is no going back once that conclusion has been reached. As the saying goes we cannot unring a bell. We are ready to take certain steps.

Step One

The steps of AA have been copied by a myriad of programs since its inception. Working the steps is a phrase that is commonly heard in these programs. Here, we are not simply copying the steps of AA. We are speaking of steps in a problem solving approach and where concepts of the venerable AA program or our interpretation of them are deemed appropriate we make use of them. It is common AA lore to say that we should do first things first. Then we work what is known as the first step.

When we look at the definition of sugar addiction the obvious first step is to stop taking in sugars in their concentrated forms. There is a slight modification of this from Section 1. We stop taking in the bad sugar. That means that we stop taking in common table sugar or cooking sugar and we stop taking in HFCS. There are two problems with making this decision. One of the problems is accurately detecting sugar. Sugars are everywhere and yet sugars are also hidden from us. It is just a fact that over time it has taken more and more sugar to give us the sweetness that we desire. Great discipline and detection skills are required to get the job of avoiding sugars done. Effort must be spent to become resensitized to an ordinary level of sweetness.

Here is a very practical example. A man in his seventies came to realize that his favorite dessert was apple pie. His mother had made apple pie for him when he was a child. His preference for the dessert had never faltered. When he ordered commercially prepared apple pies he could not mistake that the pies he bought were becoming sweeter and sweeter. When he looked at the food label on the pies that he bought he was appalled at seeing that the pies were heavily loaded with HFCS and other sugars. What was he to do?

His skills at being his own personal scientist came in handy. He decided to test the idea that it was actually apple pie that his mother had made so well in his youth. The food store was offering a pie made of apples and a whole lot of sugar. When his wife made him a pie from apples and no other sweetener he found that the pie was quite delicious. His procedure allowed him to find the taste that he had enjoyed so much in the first place. His mother had made pies for him during WWII when sugar was both very expensive and rationed. The natural sucrose, glucose and fructose combination found in apples provided all of the sweetness that the pies needed. Making apple pies without adding sugars made the more subtle taste of apple varieties available. The apples were not a vehicle for conveying sugar but were sources of satisfying taste themselves. There is no reason to believe that this sort of discovery would be limited to enjoying apple pie. Being one's own personal scientist pays off quite reliably.

This application of CBT to achieve ERFYH and deal with sugar addiction reminds us of the La Rochefoucauld admonition that to eat intelligently is an art. Any art involves the cultivation of skills. Art requires creative thinking also. We are fortunate that CBT functions as a tool that increases creative problem solving. By the time we have assessed our attitude systematically, defined the problem, considered many solutions, chosen a solution, implemented the solution, and assessed its outcome, our chances of success are very good. The goal of ERFYH has come within reach.

The temptation to turn to common artificial sweeteners as part of the problem solving has to be resisted. There is growing evidence that some so called artificial sweeteners can be harmful themselves and that they can mimic the addictive nature of sucrose and HFCS. There is no unequivocal proof of this as yet but it is prudent to operate "as if" there were. There is no need to turn to artificial sweeteners when the sort of solution demonstrated above with apple pie can be found.

Step Two

This step requires that we develop an alternative view of sugar. The method for doing that was given in the evaluation of attitude in an earlier chapter. Begin with assessing what we know about sugar and then determine what perception of it serves our purpose. For many it is helpful to follow the AA model for recovery and apply two fundamental ideas. The first of these is that we are powerless over the substance to which we are addicted. The second is that we will need the supplemental power of the God of our understanding in order to recover from that addiction. There is another way of looking at this. We can agree that we are powerless over the substance once it is in our body. We are not powerless over substances that we have not ingested. We are quite able to exercise power over the substance and throw it into the garbage.

Our present purposes require that step two must work regardless of the religious belief of the addicted person. The supplemental power that we accept for present purposes is the power of a method of problem solving that has proved effective in a wide variety of situations. It is the power of CBT when coupled with ERFYH. We leave the issue of a God of our understanding entirely up to the individual.

Those who are familiar with AA can see that we handle this matter of God's involvement just as AA did. There is no wish on our part to engage in any controversy or politics. It is up to others to argue whether CBT is a gift of God or the invention of man. For our purposes it is sufficient to recognize that CBT is the best researched therapy in use today. It has proven to be effective in a wide variety of situations including weight loss. It is a method of therapy with which we are very experienced.

Let us reframe the idea that we are powerless over "bad" sugar and are doomed to suffer from atherosclerosis. The way that we do this should seem familiar from foregoing chapters. We begin with the fact that man existed on earth for millennia before he discovered cane and beet sugar and he existed many more years before developing a way to concentrate it. It is clear from these facts that the human body does not require sugar in order to function. This is because we can make ample sugar (glucose) that our body needs from certain amino acids, using the alanine-glucose cycle or pathway. Our brains and muscle cells have priority for use of this glucose. Any change over to this pathway should be accomplished slowly to avoid excessive ketoacidosis.

Glucose differs from oxygen without which we cannot survive. Certain biological mechanisms will be triggered if we hold our breath to deprive ourselves of oxygen. We will do what is necessary to breathe. We must have oxygen. Glucose is not a must. We can say confidently that glucose is a choice. None of us are in danger of perishing from sugar deprivation.

Returning to our method for assessing attitude we can ask ourselves what sugar provides that makes it so desirable. What motivates us? There is no doubting that it gives us a taste of sweetness. There is no doubting either that there is no taste that we must satisfy in order to live. It is clearly a fact that experiencing sweetness is a choice. It is a choice that we make out of a belief that may or may not be accurate. That belief is that sugar enhances our lifestyle. Does it?

We now have the opportunity to apply a specific CBT technique to a problem of achieving ERFYH. We have described that technique before. We are speaking of being one's own personal scientist. We have already begun this process by stating the belief that is to be tested. Is it true that sugar enhances our lifestyle? We recommend that the reader write down that question.

According to our model we now collect evidence. Choose the simplest of the methods for doing this. Write down every reason that you can think of that supports the belief. It may be useful to begin with a statement such as sweet things have a pleasant and satisfying taste. Write down every one of these positive statements that come to you.

Next we write down everything that we can think of that does not support that belief. We might write down the fact that sugar is span of life and quality of life threatening. Sugar (specifically fructose) leads to atherosclerosis. We may also write that excess use of sugar can lead to obesity which obesity may then lead to many undesirable consequences such as requiring more insulin than our pancreas can generate.

Having stated the belief to be tested and listed the pros and cons that support or do not support the belief (collected evidence) we are ready to make a decision. Based on the evidence that has been collected what does it look like? What is most likely?

It is now time to implement the decision. Almost everyone needs a tip about just how to make this work. It is possible for one to change behavior instantly but usually that does not happen. Most of us need to change our behavior rather gradually. This should trigger a memory of something that we did earlier in ERFYH. A proven way to do this is to behave "as if." We take on the role of a person who has made the decision to change and has changed. We play that role much as an actor might take on the role of a Shakespearean character such as Hamlet. We will find that we receive the rewards due to a person who has genuinely decided to implement the decision that his evaluation of the collected evidence dictated. We have not truly earned those rewards but we get them anyway and they affect us.

We will begin to receive the positive remarks and admiration of peers. They will comment about our no longer using sugar in our cooking while still producing tasty meals. Significant others and our bathroom scales will notice that we are losing weight. The lab tests from our medical doctor will indicate changes in our lipid profile and fasting blood glucose level. We will see a different person in the mirror. What we will see is a person who is closer to the ideal weight for one's height. We will become the person that we are acting "as if" we were. We will no longer receive those glances that signal bewilderment that we would take in so much sugar. We will become skilled at reading food labels and making decisions on the basis of them. We will find ourselves shopping mostly in the outside walls of supermarkets as Michael Pollan recommends and we will be spending very little time in the inside rows of supermarkets where the food-like substances and processed foods are found.

We will find it useful to record evidence from our period of behaving "as if" just as we collect and record evidence in order to get started. Record the evidence at least in code. Be certain that you know exactly what role you have enacted and that you know it in detail. This evidence will speak for itself more and more as time goes by.

Too easy?

Perhaps this will sound too easy or too good to be true. Many readers will be able to look back on scores of techniques and secrets of weight control or weight loss that proved too much for them. Don't be concerned about this. ERFYH definitely is not too good to be true.

It is useful to think of the addiction process as fighting for its very survival. Every mental mechanism that there has ever been will come to the fore and interfere with recovery. We have all heard of them at one time or another. The terms include rationalization, denial, projection, and the like. Our experience indicates that it is best to regard these processes as mental cancers. They can be identified very simply. They all lead to using the addictive substance again. In this case it is sugar but the same mechanisms haunt every form of recovery. The critical idea is that they are entities produced by our mind that aim to destroy our mind. They are frankly malignant.

Regarding sugar as not harmful to us flies in the face of the fact that sugar is at the root cause of atherosclerosis and atherosclerosis is a killer. There is no evidence to support the alternative view that "bad" sugar is good for us. Nor is there evidence that "bad" sugar helps one to wind down. Sugar is as harmful in one situation as it is in another.

This brings us to another key requirement of CBT that may be remembered. That is, we must become rigorously honest with ourselves. It is not necessary to be honest with anyone else let alone be honest with everyone. It is only necessary that we be rigorously honest with ourselves. Whatever the evidence is, we must record it. If there is a "slip" and sugar is ingested in some form, we must record that. It is vital evidence. The slip can be analyzed and the vulnerability can be revealed.

Here is what we do with the evidence about a slip. We ask what it tells us about us. What was it that we believed at the time we relapsed from our program of sucrose and HFCS avoidance? Had we come to believe that "a little bit will not matter?" Had we come to believe that the process of developing atherosclerosis was not as experts told us it was? [63] For sure our behavior tells us that we had come to believe something other than what we had been taught about atherosclerosis. What were we told? Once we are certain that we have discovered the unwarranted belief we must record it. We must not let it be forgotten. For ERFYH to work we must be honest with ourselves. We must accept that the faulty belief was an honest belief that led to action. To head off the action we must head off the belief that leads to it.

What about the belief itself? It is time to evaluate the belief. How valid is it? What is the evidence pro? What is the evidence con? Which view has the weight of evidence? Which view should be made a part of the role that we will take on for the rest of our life? Which view should become a part of this new character himself?

The actions that we have just described are very clearly the most difficult of the process of coping with sugar addiction. Yet, they are the most crucial. They are the most crucial because they establish the merits of a lifestyle that is honest. It is very much along the lines of our recommendation to allow the bathroom scales to be the arbiter of whether one did or did not comply with ERFYH. The act removes this question from the realm of opinion and establishes a clear fact in its place.

The good news is that with practice being rigorously honest becomes easier and later becomes automatic. AA makes this clear in one of its Twelve Steps: When we were wrong we promptly admitted it.[64] Admitting that one is wrong requires it to be known that one was wrong. Rigorous honesty with one's self is required. When one uses the method of being one's own personal scientist and uses data instead of assertions everything works well.

This general outline of solving one's problem of sugar addiction will suffice for many who have become addicted to sugar. Understanding the nature of a common substance that has been in food for most of one's life is a major step. Simply knowing how dangerous concentrations of a naturally occurring substance can be is often sufficient to cause behavior change. Knowing also that sweetness has been increased very subtly and without our knowledge can be liberating. Knowing that this degree of sweetness has made a pleasure into a danger can be very motivating. It may be enough for enlightened behavior change.

The key to all of this is recognition that one's past quest for sweetness reflects a shift from pursuing something that is natural and healthy toward developing an underlying addictive disorder. Not many will want to do that once they know what is happening. We recall an addiction specialist who once said that in all of his years of practice he had never met an alcoholic who woke up one morning and decided to go buy a fifth of bourbon and try to become an alcoholic. Becoming overweight or obese is a gradual process. Becoming addicted to sugar is also very gradual. It is one false step or choice at a time.

Power not powerlessness

A great deal of power comes from making a decision to choose ERFYH over sugar addiction. We will turn again to AA as the oldest and most successful method of dealing with alcohol addiction. In a chapter explaining how AA works there is an often misquoted statement: "If you want what we have and are willing to go to any lengths to get it, then you are ready to take certain steps that are suggested as a program of recovery." The problem is that this emphatically is not what the book actually says. The difference is quite crucial. What the book says is: "If you have decided that you want what we have….." The absolutely critical word is "decided." Decided indicates that things have split into two or more categories and a choice has been made. The concept works only when the choice is regarded as irrevocable. Individuals come to believe that everything that has led up to the decision is now behind.

This sort of experience is common in man's history. We hear it said that the die is cast. Or, as in the case of General Dwight D. Eisenhower, on D-Day the 6th of June 1944 in WW II, the invasion was "on." There was no turning back. Successful recovery is well known to require that same view. So long as there is anything less than a decision recovery is in jeopardy.

It is a myth that nothing can be done until that decision has been made. Something very important can be done. One may begin acting "as if." In the process of acting "as if" many things can become clearer. The experience will show what it is going to be like if one makes the decision. The power of acting "as if" must not be underestimated. It is a major mechanism in CBT for ERFYH.

The decision to eliminate sweetness in its common form does not mean eliminating the pleasant experience of sweetness that man has enjoyed for most of his existence. What it means is enjoying sweetness as it occurs naturally in fruits and vegetables and rejecting manufactured concentrated sweetness. This requires some retraining but that retraining certainly can be done. It is akin to learning to appreciate the actual taste of something like watermelon or tomato instead of lavishing salt on them. Those whom we know who have done this have discovered a much more pleasant taste. It is just a fact that food tastes are often very subtle and they are varied. It takes care to discover them.

We repeat our caution that one not attempt to use sugar substitutes or the commonly available artificial sweeteners in coping with sugar addiction. The main reason for this is that it will not work. The evidence for this is overwhelming and time should not be wasted in discovering this fact for oneself.

The other compelling reason for avoiding use of artificial sweeteners is the growing evidence that they may be harmful and not benign. There is no point in taking this risk when other options are available. Nature has provided man with ample sweetness opportunities. There is no need to augment natural sweetness in anything.

Summary

We began this chapter of Section 2 with the title: The "as if" addiction and sugar addiction: their implications for ERFYH. We made the point that not every expert agrees that food addiction is a true addiction. There is good evidence that assuming that there is such an addiction can improve the chances of achieving ERFYH. This has been documented to our satisfaction and we trust that the reader who has come with us this far is persuaded. We moved on to the more popular view that sugar is addictive. We made clear that many will argue this point. We demonstrated that applying CBT to a presumed sugar addiction will greatly enhance movement to the actions necessary with ERFYH.

It will not matter whether sugar is addictive according to some professional criterion. What will matter is that the effective techniques for treating addiction have made it possible to achieve ERFYH. That is the relevant journey. That is what our effort in working together has been about from its beginning.

2.4 *Exercise counts!* But, not the way you think it does.

We subscribe to the practice that one can lose weight eating according to ERFYH with a minimum of exercise. This is not to say that exercise, done correctly, isn't important. When done correctly, it has many reliable benefits. The excessive emphasis on exercise in many weight loss programs may actually interfere with or impede weight loss. One very clear fact that must be established in the mind of anyone attempting ERFYH is that fat needs to be eliminated from one's body. The proper role of exercise in reaching that goal must be established.

This very worthwhile goal sets us against a number of myths and false beliefs that often scuttle even the best of programs. The most pervasive and harmful myth that one faces in accepting ERFYH is that exercise really defines the quality of any program aimed at losing and controlling weight. It is almost impossible to watch an exercise program on television and not hear the message that its purpose is to lose inches, weight, or both. Exercise is invariably coupled with the promise of calorie burn that will simply melt off the pounds. Nothing could be farther from the truth.

It is also important to note that what is promised by a variant of the message no pain, no gain is at odds with being healthful. Personal trainers or fitness counselors can be observed screaming and demanding more and more effort from even grossly obese persons. Some of these obese persons are those for whom intense exercise at their weight can do physical harm to joints and ligaments. This is supposed to encourage the obese individuals to exercise intensely. The theory espoused is that by expending that painful effort one will lose weight more rapidly. The facts don't support that notion.

Severe reduction in caloric intake is usually prescribed along with physical effort and pain. This sort of diet makes one hungry almost constantly. So there is another form of pain to endure. Those who fail in the face of these prescriptions are viewed as weak and unmotivated. In some cases they are quite dramatically ruled off of the program for not trying hard enough and for not gaining the expected benefit. It is said outright or implied of an individual that he/she could have lost fat but just would not pay the price to do so. Usually friends and family just shake their heads and turn away from those who fail at weight loss.

This rejection weighs heavily on those who fail to lose weight. Friends and family may fear for their loved one but they too may buy into the idea that it is lack of motivation or character which is causing the downfall. They can't imagine the individual who has been defined as weak and unmotivated ever doing enough exercise and calorie reduction to eliminate something like 100 pounds. All is despair. Every member of the problem feels this pain but they try to keep up appearances. Strategies such as selecting clothes that try to cover the obesity are developed. Nothing really works and the pain that is experienced certainly does not lead to the sort of gain that is desired. With this psychological state one can be assured that weight gain will continue.

In the face of repeated failures to lose weight by working out and expending more calories many of the overweight and obese turn to drugs or surgery to find a rapid cure. Many others simply surrender to a lifestyle that includes being ashamed, miserable, hopeless, very fat, and growing fatter. One of our colleagues even made it part of his profession as a comic to be called the Ton of Fun. Those of us who know him well understand that he is anything but fun to himself and his family. The physical and psychological consequences of this sort of psychological surrender are enormous and occur all too often. This makes us sympathetic with those who resort to desperate measures such as experimental drugs and surgery. The truth is that these attempts simply postpone an effective effort such as ERFYH. Our research says that the route to success is ERFYH. It is not more pain.

There is also a sort of sleeper concept that those who advocate extreme exercise and very restricted diets for losing fat typically overlook. We need to consider it right here. The sleeper effect is that heavy exercise generates great hunger. That degree of hunger is not consistent with what has been produced by the actual exercise. Those who exercise to lose weight almost always eat far more than enough to compensate for their energy expenditure. Taubes [65] clearly explains why this is so.

The true role of exercise in ERFYH

The true role of exercise in ERFYH is both ancillary and extremely important. Delaying the progression of atherosclerosis and the development of NCD's such as diabetes, hypertension, kidney disorders, and stroke is best accomplished with an exercise component of the ERFYH program. Things will go better with appropriate exercise included. There can be no debate about this fact. The following tells us why.

We have to change lifestyle in order to achieve our ERFYH goal. What is lifestyle? It is the collection of habits that we have built up over all of our lives. It is the collection of habits that get us by day after day.

We human beings are creatures of habit for a very good reason. Habits permit us to do many of the necessary things of our life almost without thinking. Habits of behavior are the equivalent of other self-regulating functions of the human body. We do not have to direct our stomach to digest food. Digestion of the food we take in is handled automatically for us by an elaborate system that has evolved over several millions of years. Supplying our body with oxygen works the same way. We only have to decide whether to take a breath in very special situations such as surviving a fire or swimming under water. The process of maintaining a supply of oxygen runs itself otherwise. Making most of the important behaviors for our life habitual is efficient and useful.

Not all habits that we develop are healthful. ERFYH calls for us to establish healthful food habits. ERFYH also calls for us to establish exercise habits. There is no doubt that we can develop good exercise habits at any point in our life. Having become overweight or obese may make establishing those habits a bit more difficult. To overcome this difficulty we have to maintain perspective. ERFYH will cause weight loss to proceed apace and exercise will do the same thing with what we recommend. There will be no demands for extreme amounts of exercise in this program.

Addiction "habits"

Addictions of all sorts add a degree of difficulty to changing lifestyle. It is fair to say that failures to change lifestyle and failures to achieve abstinence from alcohol and other drugs are very frequent. Failures to follow an extreme diet or exercise program seem to be at least as frequent. We hold that the failures are due to wrong thinking. There is almost no one who has not observed an overweight or obese person dieting and failing again and again. At best we may have seen a yo-yo effect of lose and gain. This is painful to watch in others and it is even more painful to experience one's self. The thoughts and behaviors of one who is obese resemble those of chronic alcoholics. We addressed these issues above in section 2.3. We always found that alcoholics maneuver to maintain the view that they will have the final say about whether they use alcohol. It is only when alcoholics turn that decision over to a recovery program that they become abstinent. It is the same way with those who have become overweight or obese. They begin to succeed when they turn over their development of an alternative lifestyle to a comprehensive program such as ERFYH.

How exercise helps

Exercise causes us to feel better about ourselves. Exercise improves our morale. Exercise is a source of joy. To open our mind about this point we need only to look at the pure joy that children experience as they run and play. Our muscles thrive on movement. We dance. We play. We experience a sort of high or mood elevation when we do these things that are very natural for us. These statements are indisputable.

We can understand the implications of this for ERFYH simply by observing. We are in almost constant motion unless our movement is artificially restricted. When sickness prevents our movement our muscles atrophy. Even our popular songs teach us that inactivity is abnormal. "Old Rockin' Chair's Got Me" is a very sad song. The song says that something has gone out of life when inactivity grabs us and we can only sit and rock. Being overweight or obese robs us of joyful movement that sitting and munching will not replace.

It is likely that in the early stages of ERFYH we will try to cope with our loss of joy from movement by sitting more and munching more. It will not work. Professionals in the addiction field would regard this strategy as trying to do the things that will not work over and over in hopes that we will have a different outcome. It is analogous to getting in the boxing ring with Muhammad Ali at his prime and expecting not to get knocked out again. What works is treating the sitting and munching as an addiction and treating it in the way we spoke about above. It is not necessary to have scientific proof that there is a food addiction before applying ERFYH.

The truth about us is self-evident. Because we are obese we human beings may have lost movement and exercise as a source of joy. That does not mean that we are happy about the loss. ERFYH shows us the way back. By using exercise as we should, the joy can be brought back. Extreme exercise will not do it but exercise as it applies to ERFYH will do it. We have a sort of muscle wisdom in that regard.

It is fair to say that our science and our common sense alike teach us to reject the view that it is only extreme exercise along with extreme calorie restriction that will cause us to lose weight and avoid atherosclerosis. We do not at all reject the idea that exercise is important to getting rid of fat. What we reject is that it does so directly.

Rebuilding the exercise aspect of one's lifestyle not only improves morale but it also helps us to reject what has taken this joy away from us. Being overweight cost us the joy. Overeating did not replace the joy. It helps to remind ourselves that fat is killing us physically by causing atherosclerosis while it is also robbing us of a major natural source of joy in our life. Mobilizing this appropriate anger toward fat can be one basis for the motivation to change.

There is good clinical evidence for all of the psychological processes that we have been discussing. In the 1940s, the psychologist and founder of a precursor to CBT, Carl Rogers, recognized that each of us develops what he called an "ideal self."[66] This "ideal self" defines for us what we want to be. It is aspirational in nature. It is also spiritual. Doing things that move us toward our "ideal self" causes us to experience pleasure. If we move away from our "ideal self" we will experience psychological pain in the form of despair or even clinical depression. Rogers found that even small steps toward the "ideal self" were antidepressant and positively motivating. We have used this insight in developing ERFYH.

Even before we regain our proper weight by ERFYH we are provided minute by minute evidence that we are moving toward our "ideal self." Every bit of scientific evidence about learning indicates that such nearly constant positive feedback or reinforcement will strengthen new learning. It will strengthen learning a new lifestyle that features fitness and health through eating the way that is natural for us.

Students often say that we really are discussing the term morale here. Many common words in our vocabulary capture something that is not debatable about the human experience. The effects of good and bad morale on human behavior are legion and have been documented throughout history. Politics, the military, and sports provide instructive examples. When we read of these experiences and look back on our own experiences almost all of us can remember a time when we suddenly went from demoralized and beaten to feeling optimistic and potent. Common sense tells us that we could not have gone from weak to strong in a matter of seconds but it seems like that. It is a fact that something actually happened. Someone who was missing critical blocks in football started making them. Armies in full retreat have been turned around and charged to victory with newfound courage. Good morale is a real asset in ERFYH. Appropriate exercise contributes to good morale.

We once listened to a young professional who was struggling with many problems. She had experienced being overweight in her teens and early twenties. She formulated her decisions about maintaining weight this way.

"There is very little in my life that I can truthfully say I have complete control of on my own. So much depends on the decisions about me that others make. However, it is up to me, and nobody else, what I do about my weight. Every day that I maintain the weight that I want to maintain is a good day and I know that I made it that way."

It is easy to see what this person's attitude toward herself and her attitude toward her weight has come to be. ERFYH aims for everyone who practices it to feel this way.

Every coach and drill sergeant knows that there is a key to turnarounds that depends on a history of appropriate exercise. Individuals who are to be rallied do best if they are already physically fit and capable. It is a truism that one cannot do what one cannot do. Morale clearly builds on physical fitness. To reach back a little one must have something to reach back to. There has to be some sort of as yet untapped reserve. Appropriate exercise provides that reserve to human beings. One will do better in confronting the problems of being overweight and addicted if he or she is also coming closer to the "ideal self" with regard to physical fitness That "ideal self" must be a self that feels potent and capable enough. Success then builds on success and fatigue does not sabotage the process.

How much exercise is enough?

We feel that "self-efficacy" defines how much exercise is enough through the measure of self esteem. Above we spoke of the psychological importance of self esteem or more specifically of striving to actualize our "ideal self." This is very relevant to the role that exercise fills with ERFYH. The closer we come to what the psychologist Abraham Maslow termed "self actualization" the more satisfied we will be.[67] Another word for this state of mind is high self esteem. It is important to note that self esteem is a very personal feeling. One may have many achievements that others admire and give rewards for but we have to regard those achievements highly. In the face of very real achievements we may despair instead of rejoice. It is not unusual for a highly acclaimed person to experience despair and even commit suicide. We have personally known more than one very accomplished clinical psychologist who committed suicide in the depths of despair and feelings of unworthiness. What one does to experience high self esteem must be both appropriate in our society and meaningful to one's self. As one moves toward success in ERFYH exercise can help to maintain and even enhance self esteem. Exercise can be very important to ERFYH even though that exercise is neither extreme nor exhausting.

The psychological concept of "self-efficacy" is one that makes very good sense when one considers taking on both lifestyle change and addiction. "Self-efficacy" refers to the personal ability to get done what one needs to get done. Much of "self-efficacy" is tied up in skill sets. The person must have the ability to do what the situation demands. Developing "self-efficacy" is a very good reason for exercising as part of learning to eat right for one's height. To be physically capable of dealing with life on its own terms one must find a way to accomplish three things from exercising. These three things are aerobic fitness, toning, and flexibility. We will consider each of them in turn.

Aerobic fitness

One must be able to sustain movement for as long as a reasonable task requires without fatiguing and quitting. Brisk walking for 45 minutes four to five times per week is often recommended to maintain aerobic fitness. ERFYH emphasizes becoming one's own personal scientist. This means that each individual should use medical and other resources to arrive at an appropriate level of aerobic exercise. ERFYH does not pit one participant against another. Exercise in ERFYH is an individual matter.

Toning

One must have enough simple muscle strength throughout one's body to pull and lift the things that one most frequently encounters in a desired lifestyle. There must be an ample reserve for coping with unusual situations. We can imagine our ancestors unexpectedly killing large game and needing to transport it. It takes muscle to bring food the long distance to home. The muscle needs to be there when it is needed. Maintaining muscle that will never be needed and carrying it all the time is just not adaptive. Tempting as it may be we do not need to bulk up.

The degree of toning and strengthening needed varies from individual to individual. For one person a full suitcase lifted to an overhead airline baggage bin might be the most strength that the lifestyle ever requires. For another the strength to move heavy furniture routinely may be required. Hobbies and work obviously vary in muscle requirements. The sort of toning exercises that will be required in order to live life as one may desire to live it obviously will vary from individual to individual. Toning should be keyed to lifestyle not weight loss, per se. Being at a proper weight adds to one's ability to deal with physical realities of any lifestyle.

The process of losing fat makes many physical efforts more realistic. Useful exercises such as the common situp are much more profitably done if one is not fighting a lot of abdominal fat. It is also much more satisfying to do pushups if one does not have a lot of fat stored above the belt. There is also great satisfaction to be had in hiking or walking briskly. The aerobic benefit is obvious. Another factor is avoiding the psychological pain that an obese person may feel when she finds herself unable to negotiate a visit to a hospitalized friend. We mentioned an actual case of this earlier in this book.

Flexibility

Some experts opine that we begin losing flexibility and our balance reflexes in our thirties or earlier. The ability to move in the direction we choose at the speed that is required and do this routinely and without injury is an essential part of exercise. Self harm in the form of strain of back muscles impairs mobility and decreases satisfaction. Flexibility exercises help prevent this problem. Both of the authors have experienced severe back pain. We sympathize with anyone who suffers this sort of pain.

We have been very impressed with a free television show that fosters flexibility. It is available on some Public Broadcasting stations. The show's DVD's are available at very reasonable cost. We recommend that readers investigate this program. Discussing the program with one's physician before starting it is recommended. The program also recommends adapting it to one's personal level of fitness. Here is the contact information for this program.

Classical Stretch - The Esmonde Technique 3437 Stanley, Suite 100 Montreal, QC Canada H3A 1S2. Information on this program may be found also at www.classicalstretch.com

What to do until motivation comes

Building a proper role for exercise into our journey for ERFYH may bring us face to face with the difficult problem of motivation. Each of us must develop an answer to the basic question of "what to do until motivation comes?" The late Willard A. Mainord, Ph.D. developed a rather novel approach to this problem which, unfortunately, he never published. Mainord combined two concepts from AA. They were "first things first" and behave "as if." He suggested that one take on the role of a motivated person for a while and play it consistently. Mainord did not require one to be motivated. Mainord only asked that one act "as if" he were motivated much as an actor might act as if he were grieving a lost love or succumbing to a fatal bullet wound.

Applying these two concepts as Mainord proposed does not require that one wait for motivation to surface. It is only necessary that one decide what the first thing is that would be done if actually motivated and then begin doing that thing. It is not necessary to really do it. One need only go through the motions of doing it. One becomes much like an actor who may be out of sorts due to his personal life but, when on stage, pretends to be very much into the requirement of his role to be happy.

Mainord's clinical evidence from the mental health ward where he worked showed that pretending to be motivated eventually caused one to become motivated. The objective evidence for this was observable behavior. Those who pretended to be motivated actually became motivated according to any reasonable criterion. Individuals did the first thing first and then acted as if they were as they wanted to be. Mainord's colleague, hypnotist Jay Haley, and Mainord probably developed this technique at about the same time. Haley labeled this technique for self motivation an aspect of paradoxical intent.[68] Mainord and Haley were most interested in the fact that it works. One can quite confidently add this technique to the tool kit for making ERFYH successful.

In this chapter we have approached exercise from the point of view of systems theory. We have observed the truism that success builds on success. Not all of us can develop attractive looks appropriate to display at poolside through weight loss and exercise but every one of us can achieve a better level of fitness than we have now. We can be certain of reaping self esteem benefits if we do.

Summary

We should not begin exercise programs believing that we will lose body FAT only when we push our bodies to extremes. Much the opposite is true. Losing body FAT requires that our morale be realistically high enough to allow us to do what needs to be done. We must take in the macronutrients and micronutrients in the correct qualities and quantities that we need day after day. Being progressively more fit will help us to pay attention as we need to meet the requirements of being our own personal scientist. Fitness will mean that we will not be fatigued from doing ordinary activities of daily living or conducting necessary investigations.

Exercising appropriately will allow us to establish a lifestyle that supports proper nutrition and vice versa. As the late James Grier Miller taught us in his major work Living Systems[69] change in any element of a system has an effect on all other parts of the system. We saw that same thing in an earlier chapter when we discussed attitude. Here it is again. The result of proper exercise helps us to have good morale and to construct the new lifestyle that we want. Achieving this goal alone builds self esteem. We probably feel better because we have earned that feeling of well being. We are practicing the principle of rigorous honesty that is so vital to dealing with addiction and addiction like entities. Having higher self esteem due to greater "self-efficacy" makes ERFYH itself more achievable. No small part of that is being able to deal with the negativism that overweight and obese individuals encounter in our society.

The results of proper exercise permit us to have good morale, move us toward our "ideal self," and allow us to develop appropriate self esteem. We achieve self esteem that is built on a realistic assessment of who we are, what we want to do, and what we can do. The old saw puts it well. Success builds on success.

We have made clear that we don't exercise to lose weight. We exercise to build the morale and self esteem that will allow us to do the things that are necessary for delaying the development of atherosclerosis. This primarily involves our losing FAT. ERFYH is enhanced by exercise but not in the way that we might have believed at the outset of our journey. The solution is not running five miles per day and eating whatever one wishes.

2.5 Bon voyage

Most of us begin life in good health. We are able to live out our life if we have appropriate nutrition including water, sunlight, and oxygen. We must also be fortunate enough to avoid accidents and the communicable diseases that our immunities cannot handle.

The undeniable fact is that very few of us make that voyage to our predicted life span successfully. The vast majority of us will die of living. Joel Elkes, M.D. termed life the great pathogen.[70] Life is about choices. The choices that we make as we go about living can reduce the amount of time that we will live.

Another way of viewing this is that most of us begin life in good health and then begin our journey to bad health. In this book we have emphasized that if the choices we make lead to atherosclerosis they accelerate our journey to bad health. If we do not eat in the way that is right for our height we can be certain that our life will be shortened more than it would be shortened otherwise.

The real voyage

We will wager that every reader of this book began reading it at some point on the journey to bad health. In all probability the reader was struggling with overweight or outright obesity. We need to acknowledge that once either of these conditions is in place it becomes very difficult to return to a healthier voyage through life.

From our experience we can say that we know of no area of life that is not affected negatively by being overweight or obese. In earlier chapters we have explained causes for overweight and obesity and we have outlined actions that will reverse the conditions and most of their consequences. We have acknowledged that there are some consequences of being overweight or obese that cannot be corrected. Knees that have been damaged by carrying far more than the load they are able to handle will have permanent damage. Corrective surgery is usually indicated if we aim to get back some of the healthy function. But it is the case that no prosthesis, wonderful as it may be, makes us as good as new.

This book provides the way to change course and not make the full voyage to ill health. It recommends that the full capacity of modern medicine be used when it is appropriate. It also recommends that some possible medical remedies be avoided because of their risks, side effects, or unintended consequences.

For the most part our book has recommended that we use the physical and mental substances and mechanisms that are natural to us. We have recommended the macronutrients in their natural form and in their proper quantities. We have recommended that the manufactured foods and the modified natural foods be avoided. We have specifically warned of the dangers inherent in eating "good" sugar and "bad" sugar that have been concentrated to the point that their unhealthy nature is made far worse.

We have emphasized those mental mechanisms that are based in Learning Theory. The techniques of CBT are the most important of these. None of these techniques artificially modify moods or states of mind. Every positive result from these therapies is earned and permanent. Nothing can take them away.

So, the real voyage that this book is concerned with is the voyage from where the reader is now to the goal of ERFYH. Other voyages will become possible after that goal has been reached. Until the goal of ERFYH is reached we will wager that all of the other goals will continue to be very unsatisfying.

Bon voyage! See you there!

References

45. Denber, H.C.B. Personal Communication.

46. Frank, Jerome *Persuasion and Healing: A Comparative Study of Psychotherapy.* Johns Hopkins University Press, 1961.

47. James, William. *Principles of Psychology.* Holt, 1890.

48. Hoffer, Eric. *The True Believer.* 1951 (Available from Amazon Books as: Hoffer, Eric *The True Believer: thoughts on the nature of mass movements.*) Perennial Classics.

49. Descartes, Rene'. http://www.goodreads.com/author/quotes/36556.Ren_Descartes

50. Descartes, Rene'. http://www.goodreads.com/author/quotes/36556.Ren_Descartes

51. Mowrer, O.H. *Learning Theory and the Symbolic Processes.* Wiley, 1960.

52. Wright, Jesse H. and Aaron T. Beck. Personal communication. 1979.

53. Elkes, Joel. Personal communication. 1976.

54. de la Rochefoucald, Francois.. In: Blackmore, A.M and Francine Gigui *Collected Maxims and Other Reflections.* Oxford World Classics, 2008.

55. Wolpe, Joseph M.D. *Psychotherapy by Reciprocal Inhibition.* Stanford University Press, 1958.

56. *Alcoholics Anonymous.* Alcoholics Anonymous Publishing Company, 1958.

57. Barrett, C. L., & Drogin, Eric "Pathological Gambling: addiction without substance." In C. D. Bryant (Series Ed.) & C. E. Faupel & P. M. Roman (Vol. Eds.), *Encyclopedia of Criminology and Deviant Behavior: Vol. 4. Self-Destructive Behavior and Disvalued Identity.* (pp. 344-346). Taylor & Francis , 2000.

58. Skinner, B.F. *The Behavior of Organisms.* Appleton–Century-Crofts, 1938.

59. James, William. *Principles of Psychology.* Holt, 1890.

60. Pollan, Michael. *The Omnivore's Dilemma.* Penquin Books, 2006.

61. Pollan, Michael. *In Defense of Food.* Penquin Books, 2008.

62. Pollan, Michael. *The Omnivore's Dilemma.* Penquin Books, 2006.

63. Esselstyn, Caldwell B., Jr., M.D. *Prevent and Reverse Heart Disease.* Penguin Group: Avery, 2007.

64. *Alcoholics Anonymous.* Alcoholics Anonymous Publishing Company, 1958.

65. Taubes, Gary. *Why We Get Fat And What To Do About It.* Knopf, 2011.

66. Rogers, C.R. *Client Centered Therapy.* Houghton Mifflin, 1951.

67. Maslow, A.H. *Motivation and Personality.* Harper, 1954.

68. Haley, Jay. *Strategies of Psychotherapy.* Grune & Stratton, 1963.

69. Miller, James G. *Living Systems.* McGraw Hill Companies, 1978.

70. Elkes, Joel M.D. Personal communication, 1976.

Epilogue

*T*he authors assume, if the reader is still with us at this point, that you have read the foregoing text in its entirety. We hope you agree with us; that is to say, something must be done to reduce fructose consumption nationally. We have toyed with many ideas but our thinking has always come back to the notion that federal and state agencies must force the removal of fructose from sucrose or table sugar and from HFCS where both commercial and domestic uses are concerned in food preparation. In addition, there should be no fructose substituted in commercially processed foods in the form of honey, maple syrup and molasses. There is nothing wrong with just providing glucose; here, it is only an issue of how much one eats, not whether, as is the case with fructose either as sucrose or HFCS. When Karo Corn Syrup first came on the market years ago, it was billed as corn syrup (and still is) which means that it contains only glucose derived from corn starch. It's an ideal sweetener; it could even be crystallized to ease dispensing. It's just hard to find it on the grocery shelf today because sucrose and HFCS have taken the market. We are confident that fructose in sucrose can be separated from glucose enzymatically to provide a fructose source for ethanol to fuel vehicles and, separately, a glucose source to fuel humans.

There is an effort afoot by food processors to call any sugar arising from corn, "corn sugar", which would further muddy the waters where food labeling is concerned. Fortunately, the FDA just denied this request for change. We also know for sure that fructose can be eliminated easily from HFCS. Just don't enzymatically convert any of the glucose of corn starch to fructose in the first place, as is currently being done. Or, if HFCS is made, make sure it is used to generate ethanol to fuel vehicles, not humans, even though ethanol from corn is clearly not a "green" process where fueling vehicles is concerned. Moreover, it is not likely to be a sustainable process as, in time, it will vastly over compete with the human need for grain. The making of ethanol from corn is already impacting grain prices, reducing grain availability vital to human consumption in poor nations as well as for the poor in the U.S. We recognize that removing fructose from these two major food sources will decrease caloric availability; that will be good for those who are overweight or obese. If slender and weight loss is not desired, one can carefully add more starch (glucose) to his/her diet to help off-set any weight loss. Grain must be used to feed humans in a sensible fashion through the use of fructose-free corn starch and fructose-free table sugar as the fundamental bioenergy sources for humans.

In another 40 years or so, the world population, currently at about 7 billion, will have grown much, much larger, perhaps by as much as 2 billion. Food sources worldwide are currently also flagging because of widespread drought conditions, including here in the U.S. How long this will continue is unknown as it may reflect warming of our oceans and erratic wind and storm currents. In the future, grain sources will have to be nurtured to sustain humans, not vehicles. Over the ensuing years, common sense dictates that we return the raising of beef, dairy cattle and sheep to open pasture grazing and allow hogs and fowl free range pasturing, as well. This would markedly decrease endemic infectious diseases and grain consumption by our chief animal protein sources, such as beef, pork, sheep, and fowl. To foster such activity, perhaps we should shift farm subsidies from corn, soybeans and wheat to encourage the growing of fruits, berries, vegetables, nuts and free range livestock. Be apprised, we do advocate federal and private insurance against crop failure because of adverse weather conditions. The latter should be continued, *ad infinitum*, when massive crop failures occur, such as in the year of 2012 here in the U.S.

Alternatives to grain sources that are being developed for feeding livestock will take some of the strain off of competition between humans and animals for grain. As an example, one alternative being developed is an extract of algae which is high in protein and fat that can be made into pellets for animal feed. While green seaweed is already used as a food source by some people around the world, scientists have now identified a bacterium that can digest inedible brown seaweed to produce sugar (glucose) to form a feed stock for biofuels. Meat protein sources are now being grown in the laboratory from pork and beef stem cells and from plant cells that have been structurally altered using recombinant DNA technology to produce animal proteins that could be used to grow meat.[71] So, help is possibly on the way for us human omnivores. We only hope it is timely for the generations to come.

The outcry from the public who will say we are interfering with their right to eat what they want to eat will be a hollow cry but one supported by industry and others, we're sure. The vast majority of lay people have no knowledge of what goes on in metabolism within their bodies. They only get an inkling once the heart attack or stroke or gangrenous extremity or other NCD problem occurs but still do not make the connection to metabolism and the correct food sources. The outcry from politicians will prove equally hollow, since politicians typically don't know much about metabolism and can be easily misdirected by lobbyists who sprinkle money around. But, please appreciate, we are already being told "what" to eat but by many large corporations that continually defy defining "what" is in the "what" we eat and its impact on health.

The food changes we propose will require a focused appeal by academicians and government scientists involved in metabolic research to the politicians and heads of various state and federal departments/agencies to do something about the issue of fructose. We only hope they are both willing to do so and prove effective in doing so. We already control alcohol, a recognized toxin, the best we can. We did learn from the debacle known as prohibition how to do this. You will notice that we say nothing here about restricting the personal use of honey, maple syrup and molasses available at the grocery; all are high in fructose and people can still get access to excessive fructose that may harm them. Molasses is a byproduct of processing sucrose; the construct of molasses may change to be only glucose with the sucrose processing we recommend. But, remember, it is one thing to have to seek out a food, it is another to have foods constantly placed before one that contain hidden sugars, particularly fructose, in amounts unknown. Moreover, we encourage the eating of fruits and berries that always contain fructose at low levels, along with vegetables that may contain some minimal amount of fructose but mostly glucose in the form of starch. Such foods are healthful for many reasons.

So, it is not like we are recommending zero fructose availability, a faulty measure reminiscent of alcohol prohibition. We have made the point that fructose turned loose on society may be causing habituation or addiction on a massive scale. But, people can get over this. Just remember, humanity survived for hundreds of thousands of years on no more than the fructose found in fruits and berries or the occasional bee hive up in a tree.

There must be regulation of the processed food industry, in addition to our many chain eateries and super markets, to achieve elimination of fructose from sweeteners used in processed foods. Fructose is clearly used to manipulate taste; it even shrouds the salty taste of restaurant food where excessive addition of salt is practiced. Fiber is reduced in processed foods to minimize water content that the bacteria need in order to thrive; fiber is an important health promoting factor. This is one reason to eat fruits and berries. There are probably other, far saner ways to control shelf life and these should be explored, if this is actually needed in today's modern food factories. As indicated earlier, it is equally important to eliminate fructose from home sweeteners. Glucose is sweet enough; we don't need fructose for additional sweetening. Remember, refined sucrose or table sugar has only been around for about 600 years (on any major scale worldwide only since modern farm equipment and techniques became available) and HFCS has been around for only about 35 years. Since we humans came down out of the trees about 2.6 million years ago, we can assume we still have the same genes that developed in ancient man to put up with the inconsistency of his food supply when he was a hunter-gatherer. Suffice it to say, we don't need to store much fructose as fat if there is no famine. This is why fruits, berries and vegetables are adequate for our need.

We think that if the above ideas involving fructose are adopted, over time, there would no longer be a physician shortage. The current providers of healthcare may not like the idea, but we could probably close some of our medical schools, hospitals and clinics. These are all factors on the expense side of the ledger sheet. This offers a way to reduce cost and provide healthcare on reasonable financial terms. Medication consumption would be reduced drastically. A national incidental *pro bono* weight loss program would occur for most who need it without any other intervention by the individual. This would be in contradistinction to almost all participatory weight loss regimens that generally fail long term and would not ever be feasible on the vast scale required to arrest growth in the medical issues confronting our entire nation. One would have to be extremely naïve to believe that over 200 million people will willfully adopt a proper low fructose diet to restore them to an ideal body weight to avoid or mitigate atherosclerosis. Exercise counts in health but proper food intake counts much, much more in maintaining a healthful weight. Exercise is not a requirement for weight loss but it is a requirement for maintaining muscle strength and brain and cardiovascular health. Starch remains an excellent source of glucose; again, here, it is only an issue of how much, not whether, in the making of body fat. We really don't need industrially produced sucrose or HFCS in our food supply.

What we have described provides one sure way that, over time, Medicare and Medicaid can be brought onto a fiscal trajectory workable for the long haul. Why would this happen? Well, just think about it: There would eventually be a major reduction in clinical vascular disease, particularly in the middle aged and elderly populations and there would be a corresponding reduction in all the bad health baggage over and above atherosclerosis that is incumbent to what we currently eat, young or old. It is estimated that about 76 million baby boomers will be retiring and seeking Medicare coverage over the next two decades, so we had better do something to lower medical costs.[72] In our opinion, limiting fructose is the only sensible way to limit the inexorable growth of the NCD portion of medical costs in a reasonable and reliable manner. And, removing industrially produced fructose from the food supply is one accomplishable with only some one time costs plus tradeoffs in costs. That is, glucose from sucrose would be a little more expensive due to the need for enzymatic treatment and separation of fructose, while glucose from corn starch would be a little less expensive by getting rid of the enzymatic treatment to produce HFCS in the first place.

One just has to remember that the CHO's (fructose and alcohol for sure and glucose if eaten excessively) are what trigger DNL in the liver that produces

VLDL that leads to excess oxidized LDL, the so-called "bad" CHOL, a causative factor of atherosclerosis. One should also remember that LDL is a nanoparticle comprised of four principal things – a PROT rod with attached PL, TRIG and CHOL All can be oxidized. Referring to LDL as LDL CHOL is an archaic hold over term from days past; it only tends to confuse issues relevant to CHO metabolism and health and disease. It surely confuses the public about what is important in one's diet and perhaps some academicians as well. Why not just call it what it is? Call it LDL nanoparticles.

Finally, we see no vast economic impediments to adopting elimination of fructose in processed foods or eliminating its use in the home; in fact, we see only emotional impediments. Considering all of the NCD's that accompany excess CHO intake, particularly that of fructose, this move would improve substantially one's "health span" within one's theoretical "life span" of 120 years. Because of growth in population numbers in coming years, we must anticipate even greater availability of both processed foods and artificially constructed "foods". This will elevate the need to control fructose use commercially to an even greater degree. Atherosclerosis does not have to be destiny; one just has to learn how to feed one's physiology correctly and health will be at his/her back.

References

71. Bartholet, J. "Inside the Meat Lab." *Scientific American* (June 2011). pp. 65-69.
72. Antos, Joseph R. "The Wyden-Ryan Proposal – A Foundation for Realistic Medicare Reform." *NEJM* (March 8, 2012). 366;10:879.

Appendix A

$\mathscr{F}$or those who may wish to become further acquainted with Cognitive Behavior Therapy (CBT) from the mainstream media we are providing some references to help with getting a start. These are basic texts that were developed well after the seminal work of Aaron T. Beck, M.D. on CBT of Depression. The reader will notice that CBT has matured since the early work in the field and today the Academy of Cognitive Therapy (of which Dr. Barrett is a Founding Fellow) represents that maturity. The reader should note that today the term Cognitive Therapy (CT) is commonly used. Our use of the term is the one we were used to in the field's formative days: Cognitive Behavior Therapy. This term recognizes the fact that many psychologists found the addition of cognitive to the learning theory approaches of the time known as Behavior Therapy quite satisfying. The idea of the human being as a Black Box was never satisfying to Clinical Psychologists as group but the rigor of Behavior Therapy and its clear results with difficult patients provided psychologists with useful therapeutic tools that were not available in the late 1950s. The marriage of Behavior Therapy and Cognitive Therapy has all but revolutionized the field of psychotherapy. We believe that the following readings will intrigue those who seek ERFYH.

Beck, Judith S. *The Beck DIET Solution.* Oxmoor House. 2007

Burns, Robert *Feeling Good: The New Mood Therapy* [Mass Market Paperback] 1999

Wright, J.H. & M.R. Ramirez Basco *Getting Your Life Back.* Simon & Schuster. 2001

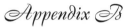

Appendix B

Form for Evaluating Attitude

In this form you are asked to answer questions about your attitude toward
_____. Bear in mind that attitude is
defined here as: *A learned, specific, predisposed way to respond to a specific set of stimuli.*

What do you KNOW about _____?
Please answer this question completely in the following area of this form.

What do you WANT from _____?
Please answer this question completely in the following area of this form.

What do you FEEL about _____?
Please answer this question completely in the following area of this form.

How do you SEE _____?
Please answer this question completely in the following area of this form.

Now, put all of the elements of your attitude toward _____
_____ together in the way that best helps you understand
how all of these components work together. For example, how does what you
know, or do not know, affect how you "see" _____?

Now that you know the anatomy of YOUR attitude toward _____
_____, do you want to change the attitude
or leave it as it is? *Write* your answer to this question explaining your decision.

How do you feel now that you have made the decision to keep or to change your
attitude toward _____?

Index

A

ab luminal atheromata, 47

abetalipoproteinemia, 42

Academy of Cognitive Therapy, 151

acetaldehyde, 21, 25

acetic acid, 22, 54

acetyl-CoA carboxylase-1 (ACC-1), 16, 20

acetyl-CoA synthetase, 22

acute coronary syndromes, 5, 47

ad luminal atheromata, 47

addiction

    "as if" addiction and, 98, 103-107, 118, 121, 123-124, 127-128, 138

    coping with sugar addiction, 110-111

    fundamentals of treating and, 101-103

    "habits" and, 132

    sugar addiction and, 98, 116-117, 119-124, 127-128

    understanding and, 98-101

adenosine tri-phosphate (ATP), 10, 18-20, 33, 36, 41

adenosine tri-phosphate citrate lyase (ACL), 16, 20

aerobic fitness, 136

alcohol

    calories and, 22

    control of, 147

    DNL in the liver and, 149-150

    FAT masquerading as CHO and, 34

    management of, 21-23

    negative physiologic impacts of, 25-27

alcohol dehydrogenase-1B, 21

Alcoholics Anonymous (AA), xxviii, 94, 99-100, 102, 105, 120-122, 126-127, 138

alcoholism, fundamentals of treating addiction and, 92, 99, 101-102

aldehyde, 18, 21-22, 25, 44-45

aldehyde dehydrogenase-2, 22

aldosterone, 59

Ali, Muhammad, 133

alkalinity, 51

Ampulla of Vater, 12

Ampulla's Sphincter of Oddi, 12

angiotensin-II, 59

anti-oxidants, 50

antigout medications, 49

antihypertensives, 49

Apo B-100 PROT, 15, 22-23, 38, 42

apocalypse, xxviii, 7, 67-68

apoptosis, liver and nerve cell death, 25

apoptotic, cell death and, 40, 50

apple pie, 56, 120-121

arterial plaques, 6, 40, 69

artificial sweeteners, 121, 128

"as if" addiction, 98, 103-107, 118, 121, 123-124, 127-128, 138

aspirin, xiv, 9, 49

assumptive world, 79-80

atheroma, xxvii-xxviii, 40, 46-50, 66

atheromata

    formation of, 46-48

    minimizing atheromata formation and, 48-49

    atheromatous, arteries containing atheromata and, xxviii, 47-49

atherosclerosis

    acute coronary syndromes and, 5, 47

    cardiovascular disease and, 5, 8, 49, 65, 67

D

dehydrogenase-1B, 21

de La Rochefoucauld, Francois, 87, 98, 121

Denber, Herman C.B., 77

de novo lipogenesis (DNL)

> chylomicrons and, 11, 37, 39, 64
>
> concept of fractional DNL and, 27-30
>
> conversion to fatty acids and, 15-16, 18, 23-24, 64
>
> dietary intake of FAT and, 34-36
>
> "lipid droplet" problem and, 30-32
>
> management of alcohol and, 21-22
>
> management of glucose and, 19-20
>
> negative physiologic impacts of alcohol and fructose, 35
>
> overview of, xxvii
>
> proclivity to form fat and, 10
>
> production of LDL CHOL and, 69
>
> production of ROS in the liver and, 45, 149-150

dendritic cells, 6, 45, 47

denial, 125

Descartes, Rene, 80-81, 83

Detroit Marathon (2009), 7-8

diabetes

> blood glucose levels and, 45
>
> excessive endopic and ectopic lipogenesis, 55
>
> exercise and, 131
>
> hyperlipidemia and, 29
>
> irreversible pancreatic beta cell damage and, 37
>
> management of alcohol and, 21
>
> non-communicable diseases (NCD's) and, 77, 131
>
> nonalcoholic fatty liver disease (NAFLD) and, 31, 37

obesity and, 83

> sugar addiction and, 109
>
> sugar cane and, 110
>
> type 2 diabetes mellitus (T2DM) and, xxiii, 13, 35, 61, 114

diapedesis, 5-6

diet

> alcohol consumption and, 52
>
> Atkins' Diet and, 55
>
> Atwater caloric values and, 22, 52
>
> avoid excessive ketoacidosis and, 53-54
>
> caloric intake per macronutrient and, 51-52
>
> controlling inflammation and, 54
>
> controlling macronutrient proportions and, 52
>
> controlling one's metabolism and, 53-54
>
> eating properly chosen nuts and, 53
>
> grazing and, 116-117
>
> ideal body weight and, 51, 54, 149
>
> moderate starch (glucose) consumption and, 52-53
>
> more discussion on, 54-60
>
> normal kidney function and, 55-56
>
> optimize body weight and, 51
>
> optimizing PROT intake and, 53
>
> rationale for targeted therapy and, 60-69
>
> reducing LDL nanoparticle numbers and, 50-54
>
> restricting fruit and certain vegetable consumption and, 52
>
> sugar addiction and, 119-124, 127-128

dihydroxyacetone-P, 18-19, 45

Disappearance Data (2010), per capita intake of sugar and, 21

distance runners, 7-9

diuretics, 58

DNA, cellular gene structure within nucleus and, 16, 46, 147

docosahexaenoic acid (DHA), 6

double column technique, 87

Drogin, Eric, 102

E

F

gambling addiction, 102

glow worms, New Zealand Cave and, 83, 109, 111

glucagon, 13, 35

gluconeogenesis, 13, 17, 35-36

glucose

    alanine-glucose cycle and, 122

    aldehyde form in the liver and, 45

    apple pies and, 121

    "bad" CHOL and, 39-40

    blood-borne glycation of proteins and, 44-45

    "carb loading" and, 9

    case study and, 114

    chylomicron levels and, 64

    converted to fatty acids and, 10

    corn syrup and, 26, 112, 145

    diet construction and, 51

    DNL in the liver and, 149-150

    early recovery point for, 12

    exercise and, 124

    fatty acid conversion products of DNL
        and, 23-24

    fractional DNL and, 27-30, 36

    glucose-alanine cycle and, 56

    high fructose corn syrup (HFCS) and, 109

    impact on insulin and, 32-33

    insulin resistance and, 35

    insulin secretion and, 34

    Karo Corn Syrup and, 145

    ketosis and, 54-55

    Krebs Cycle and, 22

    LDL production and, 50

    management of, 19-20

    minimizing atheromata formation and, 48-49

    moderate starch (glucose) consumption
        and, 52-53

    molasses and, 147

    obesity and, 60, 67

    off-setting weight loss and, 146

    overview of, xv-xvi, xxiv-xxvii, 100

    per capita intake of, 21

    production of insulin and, 13

    production of LDL CHOL and, 69

    spices and herbs, 57

    storage in the liver and, 11

    sugar addiction and, 108

    sweetness of, 148

    synthesis of VLDL and, 15-17

    weight loss and, 37

glucose transporters (GLUT), 12, 16-17, 19, 25-26

GLUT-2, 19

GLUT-3, 19

GLUT-4, 12, 19

GLUT-5, 16-17, 25-26

glycation, xxvii, 11, 18, 21, 25, 40, 44-45

glyceraldehyde-3-P, 18-19, 45

glycogenolysis, 13, 35-36

"God of our understanding", 121-122

grains, 146-147

grazing, 117-119

$\mathcal{H}$

habits, addictive and, 132

Haley, Jay, 138

HDL CHOL, 30, 63

Health and Human Services Department, 26

health span, 55, 150

heart attacks, xxiii, 5, 48, 67

hemoglobin, 44

HemoglobinA1c, 44

HgA1C test, 114

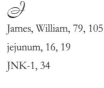

"ten year heart attack risk calculator", 66-67

Thanksgiving Day 10k Race (2010), 8

Think System (*Music Man* idea), 80-81, 85-88

threshold, for taste of salt and, 59

thyroid stimulating hormone (TSH), 62

Ton of Fun, 130

toning, 136-137

triathlon, New York Triathlon (2011), 8

triglyceride (TRIG)

    Apo-B100 PROT rod and, 22

    B100 PROT rod and, 19

    chylomicrons and, 36-39

    effects of ROS during metabolism and, 18

    family related risk factors for atherosclerosis and, 63

    fatty acids and, 24-25, 42

    HSL's intracellular action and, 36

    LDL nanoparticleas and, 69, 150

    "lipid droplet" problem and, 30-32

    lipogenesis and, 33-36

    NEFA's storage capacity for, 34

    oleic acid and, 20, 23-24

    overview of, xxvii

    post-prandial hypertriglyceridemia and, 29

    reconversion of fatty acids to, 10, 12, 33

    reversing CHOL transport and, 49-50

    synthesis of VLDL and, 15

    targeted therapy and, 63-65

The True Believer (Hoffer), 79

Twelve steps, Alcoholics Anonymous (AA) and, 99, 126

type 2 diabetes mellitus (T2DM), xxiii, 13, 35, 61, 114